MAGNETIC RESONANCE IMAGING OF BONE AND SOFT TISSUE TUMORS AND THEIR MIMICS

SERIES IN RADIOLOGY

Volume 20

1. J. Odo Op den Orth, The Standard Biphasic-Contrast Examination of the Stomach and Duodenum: Method, Results and Radiological Atlas.
   1979. ISBN 90 247 2159 8
2. J.L. Sellink and R.E. Miller, Radiology of the Small Bowel. Modern Enteroclysis Technique and Atlas.
   1981. ISBN 90 247 2460 0
3. R.E. Miller and J. Skucas, The Radiological Examination of the Colon. Practical Diagnosis.
   1983. ISBN 90 247 2666 2
4. S. Forgács, Bones and Joints in Diabetes Melitus.
   1982. ISBN 90 247 2395 7
5. G. Németh and H. Kuttig, Isodose Atlas. For Use in Radiotherapy.
   1981. ISBN 90 247 2476 7
6. J. Chermet, Atlas of Phlebography of the Lower Limbs, including the Iliac Veins.
   1982. ISBN 90 247 2525 9
7. B. Janevski, Angiography of the Upper Extremity.
   1982. ISBN 90 247 2684 0
8. M.A.M. Feldberg, Computed Tomography of the Retroperitoneum. An Anatomical and Pathological Atlas with Emphasis on the Fascial Planes.
   1983. ISBN 0 89838 573 3
9. L.E.H. Lampmann, S.A. Duursma and J.H.J. Ruys, CT Densitometry in Osteoporosis. The Impact on Management of the Patient.
   1984. ISBN 0 89838 633 0
10. J.J. Broerse and T.J. MacVittie, Response of Different Species to Total Body Irradiation.
    1984. ISBN 0 89838 678 0
11. C. L'Herminé, Radiology of Liver Circulation.
    1985. ISBN 0 89838 715 9
12. G. Maatman, High-resolution Computed Tomography of the Paranasal Sinuses, Pharynx and Related Regions.
    1986. ISBN 0 89838 802 3
13. C. Plets, A.L. Baert, G.L. Nijs and G. Wilms, Computer Tomographic Imaging and Anatomic Correlation of the Human Brain.
    1986. ISBN 0 89838 811 2
14. J. Valk, MRI of the Brain, Head, Neck and Spine. A Teaching Atlas of Clinical Applications.
    1987. ISBN 0 89838 957 7
15. J.L. Sellink, X-Ray Differential Diagnosis in Small Bowel Disease. A Practical Approach.
    1988. ISBN 0 89838 351 X
16. T.H.M. Falke, ed., Essentials of Clinical MRI.
    1988. ISBN 0 89838 353 6
17. B.D. Fornage, ed., Endosonography.
    1989. ISBN 0 7923 0047 5
18. R. Chisin and A.L. Weber, eds., MRI/CT and Pathology in Head and Neck Tumors. A Correlative Study.
    1989. ISBN 0 7923 0227 3
19. G. Gozzetti, A. Mazziotti, L. Bolondi, L. Barbara, eds., Intraoperative Ultrasonography in Hepato-Biliary and Pancreatic Surgery. A Practical Guide.
    1989. ISBN 0 7923 0261 3

MAGNETIC RESONANCE IMAGING OF BONE AND SOFT TISSUE TUMORS AND THEIR MIMICS

A Clinical Atlas

A.M.A. DE SCHEPPER
and
H.R.M. DEGRYSE

*Department of Radiology,
University Hospital Antwerp, Belgium*

with contributions by

F. De Belder
L. van den Hauwe
F. Ramon
P. Parizel
N. Buyssens

KLUWER ACADEMIC PUBLISHERS
DORDRECHT / BOSTON / LONDON

ISBN-13: 978-94-010-6938-0   e-ISBN-13: 978-94-009-0997-7

DOI:10.1007/ 978-94-009-0997-7

Published by Kluwer Academic Publishers,
P.O. Box 17, 3300 AA Dordrecht, The Netherlands.

Kluwer Academic Publishers incorporates
the publishing programmes of
D. Reidel, Martinus Nijhoff, Dr W. Junk and MTP Press.

Sold and distributed in the U.S.A. and Canada
by Kluwer Academic Publishers,
101 Philip Drive, Norwell, MA 02061, U.S.A.

In all other countries, sold and distributed
by Kluwer Academic Publishers Group,
P.O. Box 322, 3300 AH Dordrecht, The Netherlands.

PREFACE

Magnetic resonance imaging has already become a most valuable imaging modality in the diagnostic work-up of musculoskeletal neoplasms. While high accuracy of MRI for staging purposes has been proven, we will focus in this monograph on the characterization of primary bone and soft tissue tumors by MRI.

The major purpose of this monograph is to provide an atlas of magnetic resonance features of primary bone and soft tissue tumors for radiologists, orthopedic surgeons and physiotherapists.

The results presented are based on investigations of 94 primary bone and soft tissue tumors and mimicking conditions by magnetic resonance imaging. Although the scale of the material allows for statistical handling, the number of patients per subgroup is too small to come to definite conclusions.

We will therefore limit ourselves to the description of and comments on a great number of cases to illustrate the diagnostic potential of this new imaging modality.

We would like to thank the anonymous cooperators: referring clinicians, pathologists, nurses, technicians and secretaries whose help enabled us to present this monograph. We would also like to express our gratitude to the firms Siemens AG and Schering AG for technical support.

This monograph results from the will to do clinical-scientific research with and despite the limited manpower and infrastructure of a small but dynamic university department.

Key to abbreviations

CR	Conventional radiography
CT	Computed tomography
DSA	Digital subtraction angiography
MR	Magnetic resonance
MRI	Magnetic resonance imaging
RNSC	Radionuclide scintigraphy
SE	Spin echo
SI	Signal intensity
WI	Weighted images

CONTENTS

1 General Considerations about Bone and Soft Tissue Tumors 5
2 Materials and Methods 21

Benign Bone Tumors and Mimicking Conditions

3 Osteoid Osteoma 25
4 Enchondroma 31
5 Osteochondroma 34
6 Giant Cell Tumor 39
7 Vertebral Hemangioma 44
8 Solitary Bone Cyst 50
9 Aneurysmal Bone Cyst 52
10 Non Ossifying Fibroma 56
11 Eosinophilic Granuloma 58
12 Fibrous Dysplasia 61
13 Osteomyelitis 69

Malignant Bone Tumors

14 Osteogenic Sarcoma 75
15 Chondrosarcoma 75

Benign Soft Tissue Tumors

16 Lipoma 98
Neurogenic Tumor 99
Soft Tissue Hemangioma 102
Aggressive Fibromatosis 104

Malignant Soft Tissue Tumors

17 Liposarcoma 109
18 Malignant Fibrous Histiocytoma 115
19 Rhabdomyosarcoma 118

20 Value of Contrast (Gd-DTPA)-Enhanced MRI Studies in Cases of Musculoskeletal Tumors 123

21 General Conclusions 129

CHAPTER 1:

GENERAL CONSIDERATIONS ABOUT BONE AND SOFT TISSUE TUMORS:

1.1 INTRODUCTION:

Medical imaging and histopathology are both essential in the study of musculoskeletal neoplasms. The complementarity of both methods has been stressed to the best by R.Freiberger in his article "Thoughts on the Diagnosis of Bone Tumors" (7). Its abstract will serve as an introduction and a guide throughout the material discussed below:
'The pathologist and the radiologist have each been given reason to believe that he is capable of accurately diagnosing bone tumors without the assistance of the other. However, each specialist has recourse to tools and procedures not available to the other, and their findings should be considered as complementary. Although there are radiographic features which could be an indication of malignancy, there are too many common exceptions to formulate a general rule. Likewise, although the pathologist can examine microscopic morphology and obtain biochemical information using special stains, the sample being examined may not be representative of the entire tumor. Thus the ultimate benefit to the patient can be obtained only if the radiologist and pathologist work in concert with one another and with the surgeon toward the common goals of accurate diagnosis and prompt, appropriate management of bone tumors.'

Two cases of our series dramatically illustrate the need for a permanent confrontation of radiological and pathological data.

In the case of L.V., a 14 year-old female, clinical data as well as findings on various imaging techniques indicate the presence of an osteoid osteoma (Fig. 1.1).
Histological examination only shows 'highly compact bone layers with irregular and dilated Haversian canals: signs indicating a hyperostotic lesion.' Although clearly demonstrated by all imaging methods, the characteristic "nidus" was not visualized histologically.
The results of the radio-pathological confrontation, however, allow an almost certain diagnosis of osteoid osteoma.

A second illustrative case concerns D.P.D., a 9 year-old boy, presenting with pain in the region of the left fibula, after a sport injury (Fig.1.2). On CR a bony lesion at the fibular diaphysis is found. Despite its geographical appearance, suggesting a benign condition, no sclerotic margins are recognized and there is a slight disruption in the periosteal new bone formation at the medial border of the lesion (Fig. 1.2.a). On CT there is evidence of a subtle, unsharply delineated, hypodense paracortical area (Fig. 1.2.d).
On MRI, the central intramedullary lesion has a relatively high SI [4] on T1-WI (Fig 1.2.b), whereas the semilunar paracortical area has an increased SI [6] on T2-WI (Fig. 1.2.c).These findings are not consistent with a benign lesion. Because of the discrepancy between the clinical and radiological findings, the lesion has been removed surgically. Histological examination shows 'a pronounced periosteal reaction and irregular Haversian canals. The lesion itself is cystic and contains a highly proteinaceous fluid. The cyst is complicated by a concomitant pathologic fracture.
Retrospectively, these findings explain the MRI-characteristics of the lesion: the high protein concentration in the fluid shortens the T1-relaxation time and causes an increased SI. The periosteal reaction is a consequence of the pathologic fracture. The paracortical lesion on CT as well as on MRI corresponds to a non-recent hemorrhage, as reflected by the prolongation of the T2-relaxation time.

6

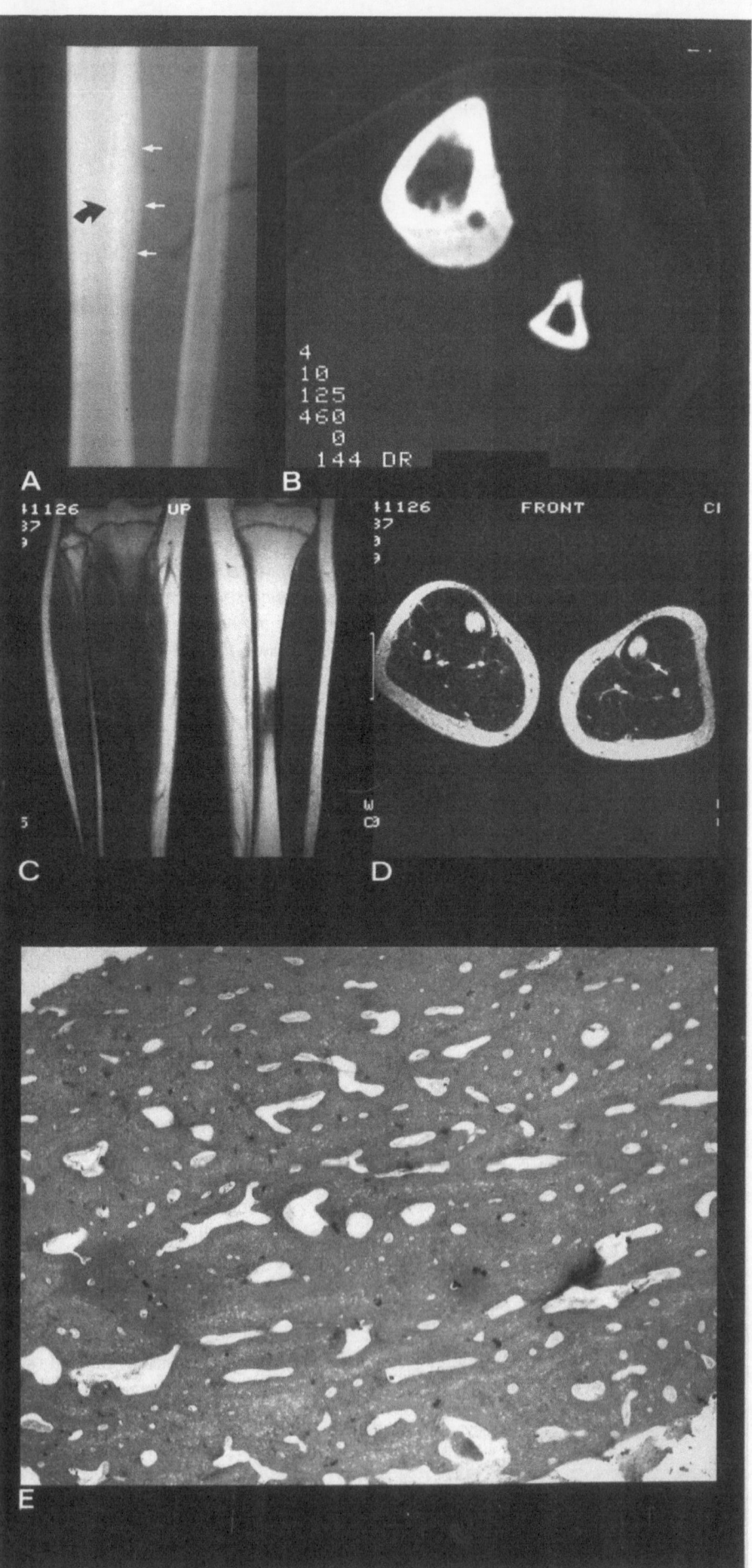

Fig. 1.1. L.V., 14 year-old female.

1.1.a. CR of the middle third of the left
    tibia. Localized cortical thickening and
    hyperostosis at the lateral border of
    the tibia (arrows). A small central
    lucent area within the hyperostotic
    region is noted (curved open arrow).
1.1.b. CT at the level of the lesion, bone
    window.
    Cortical thickening by hyperostosis
    is confirmed. The enclosed lucent
    area is clearly demonstrated.
1.1.c. MRI of the lower legs, coronal
    section, T1-WI.
    The area of hyperostosis is seen as
    a fusiform broadening of cortical signal
    void. Geographical area of decreased
    SI in the adjacent bone marrow.
1.1.d. MRI at the level of the lesion,
    transverse section, T2-WI.
    Again, cortical hyperostosis presents
    as an enlargement of the cortical
    signal void. Within it a small
    hyperintense fleck is observed (arrow).
1.1.e. Microphotograph of biopsy specimen
    (Courtesy Prof Van Damme, KUL).
    Dense osseous tissue with small
    marrow cavities. Reactive hyperplasia.
    Absence of nidus.
Diagnosis : Osteoid osteoma of the tibia.
    Although not demonstrated
    pathologically, a nidus was clearly
    shown by various imaging techniques.

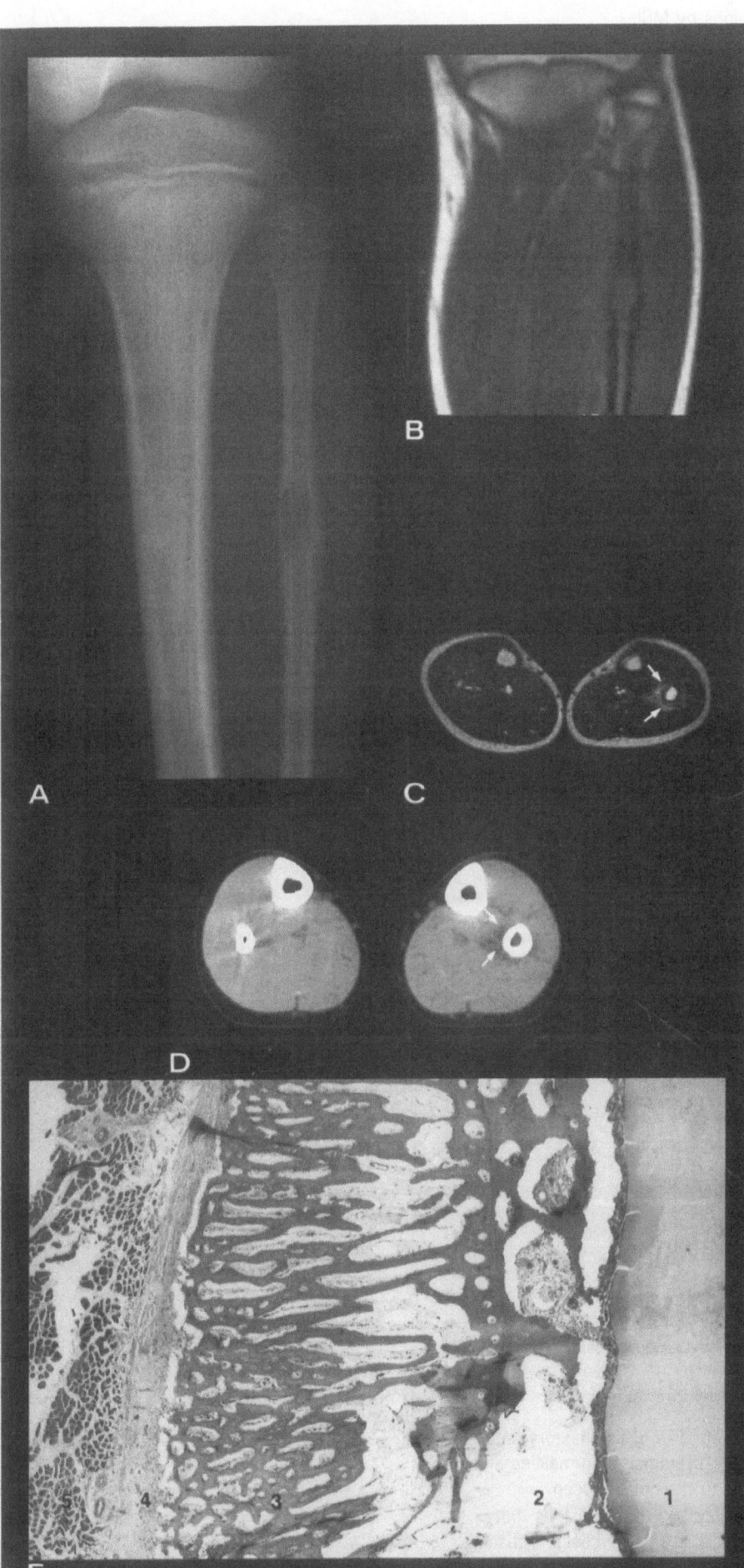

Fig. 1.2. D.P.D., 9 year-old male.

1.2.a. CR of the proximal part of the left lower leg.

Slightly expansive lesion in the proximal part of the fibular diaphysis, causing endosteal scalloping. Absence of sclerotic rim. Periosteal elevation, pronounced at the lateral fibular margin. Slight disruption at the medial border.

1.2.b. MRI of the left fibula, coronal section, T1-WI.

The intramedullary lesion presents with decreased SI [3] compared to normal bone marrow. Endosteal scalloping and periosteal reaction are also seen.

1.2.c. MRI of the left fibula at the level of the lesion, transverse section, T2-WI. Markedly raised SI of the medullary component of the lesion [7]. Moderate increased SI [6] in the adjacent muscle, posteriorly and medially to the lesion (arrows).

1.2.d. CT of the left fibula at the level of the lesion, soft tissue window. Enlargement of the medullary cavity, indicating expansive intramedullary lesion, is seen. Slight ill defined hypodense area in adjacent muscle (arrows).

1.2.e. Microphotograph. (Courtesy Prof Van Damme, KUL)

Margin of simple bone cyst:

1/ lumen,

2/ pre-existing cortical bone with pressure atrophy,

3/ new bone formation,

4/ periosteal connective tissue,

5/ striated muscle.

Diagnosis: Juvenile bone cyst, complicated by pathological fracture

Besides the importance of the radiopathological confrontation, this case already illustrates the potential of morphologic approach and of tissue characterization of bone and soft tissue lesions by MRI.

1.2 DIAGNOSTIC VALUE OF VARIOUS IMAGING TECHNIQUES:

Medical Imaging deals with *detection, definition of extent and characterization* of musculoskeletal tumors, which are all essential for adequate therapy planning.
The purpose of this study is to determine whether pertinent diagnostic information, not given by other imaging methods, can be obtained by Magnetic Resonance Imaging (MRI), being the newest imaging modality (3,18).

1.2.1 Bone tumors, detection and diagnosis:

Despite a relative insensitivity to some marrow neoplasms (lymphoma, leukemia and myeloma) and some aggressive metastatic tumors, SCINTIGRAPHY (radionuclide scintigraphy) is still a highly valuable method in the detection of bone tumors (15).

CONVENTIONAL RADIOGRAPHY and conventional TOMOGRAPHY remain most important tools for the detection and diagnostic work-up of these tumors (9). They allow an excellent appreciation of bone destruction (geographic, moth-eaten or permeative), bone reaction (with the presence or absence of a "sclerotic rim", an expanded shell or bone erosion), transition zone between tumor and adjacent normal bone and endosteal-periosteal reaction (solid, lamellated, spiculated, 'Codman's triangle').
Although the relativity of classifications is stressed by the authors themselves, we found the most reliable and simplified radiographic classification of local behaviour of bone tumors in "Radiologic Management of Musculoskeletal Tumors"(Springer Verlag, 1987) by H.Pettersson, D.Springfield and W.Enneking (14). This classification is presented in table 1.1 (by courtesy of the authors).

Table 1.1: Simplified radiographic classification of the local behaviour of bone tumors.

Local behaviour:	Radiologic characteristics:
Latent	Geographic destruction Cortical "rim" or "capsule" Expanded cortex < 1 cm, if any Solid periosteal reaction, if any
Active	Geographic destruction Thin, well-defined transition zone Thin or no cortical capsule Cortical penetration acceptable' Expanded cortex > 1 cm Solid or lamellated periosteal reaction if any
Aggressive	Moth-eaten/ permeative destruction Ill-defined transition zone No cortical capsule Cortical and periosteal penetration Lamellated or perpendicular periosteal reaction Associated soft tissue mass

Together with some other, easily evaluable data, like clinical history, sex, age of the patient, localization(s) of the lesion, systemic abnormalities and laboratory findings, one will not only be able to distinct between non-aggressive, moderately aggressive or highly aggressive lesions, but even to make an accurate histological diagnosis in a lot of cases. These methods do not require sophisticated equipment and are evenso interesting from the economic point of view.

COMPUTED TOMOGRAPHY will confirm the findings of conventional radiography and better demonstrate some of them. In addition, due to the superior inherent contrast resolution, CT will add some new data. Hence, diagnostic accuracy is improved when combining CR and CT. Furthermore, the use of Iodine-containing contrast media is indicative of the degree of vascularization of the lesion and will eventually obviate the need for angiography.

The limitation to perform uniquely unidirectional (axial) approach of the lesion, and the presence of streak artifacts (near the thick cortical bone and by metal clips or implants) are well known disadvantages of CT.

ANGIOGRAPHY will contribute only in a lesser degree to the diagnosis of bone tumors. The vascular pattern of these tumors is rarely typical for a given type of tumor and is not even a parameter for the degree of aggressiveness of the tumor. DIGITAL SUBTRACTION ANGIOGRAPHY, mostly performed by intraarterial contrast injection, has the advantage of better demonstrating a tumoral blush or abnormal vascularity, as in osteosarcoma and osteoid osteoma ('nidus').

1.2.2 Soft tissue tumors, detection and diagnosis:

In the detection and characterization of soft tissue tumors both SCINTIGRAPHY and CONVENTIONAL RADIOGRAPHY - TOMOGRAPHY are of little value.
ULTRASONOGRAPHY may demonstrate the presence of a soft tissue mass, but lacks specificity in the majority of cases.
For reasons discussed already, COMPUTED TOMOGRAPHY, performed before and after the injection of Iodine containing contrast material, will be capable to detect the tumor and to characterize it in a great number of cases (lipoma, liposarcoma, hemangioma).Besides the advantages mentioned above, a lot of soft tissue masses have CT-attenuation values similar to those of surrounding muscle, making their detection more difficult (12).
The value of CONVENTIONAL ANGIOGRAPHY and DSA in the detection and diagnosis of soft tissue tumors is comparable with that in the diagnosis of bone tumors. As a matter of fact, angiomatous lesions will be better demonstrated angiographically.

1.2.3 Bone and soft tissue tumors, evaluation of extent:

Besides its detection and diagnosis, with tissue characterization in the optimal situation, exact evaluation of the extent of bone and soft tissue tumors is a challenge for medical imaging.
SCINTIGRAPHY is able to demonstrate extent of primary bone tumors into adjacent soft tissues or bone invasion by soft tissue neoplasms but provides poor anatomic detail.
Although extent of tumor within soft tissues can be evaluated by ULTRASONOGRAPHY, intraosseous spread of tumor cannot be determined by this modality.
CONVENTIONAL RADIOGRAPHY and TOMOGRAPHY are capable of detecting osseous involvement but are relatively insensitive to the determination of extent of primary soft tissue tumors or extension of bone tumors into soft tissues (5).
Until recently, COMPUTED TOMOGRAPHY was the best imaging modality to visualize this extent. The excellent anatomic detail, the superior contrast resolution, the more exact densitometry, the better appreciation of tumor vascularization and the better demonstration of the spatial relationship between tumor, muscles, muscular compartments, fascial planes and neurovascular structures by this method are responsible for this. Although roughly demonstrated, invasion of the medullary cavity is less accurate with CT than with MRI. Controversy exists about the accuracy of CT in the assessment of tumor relationship with neurovascular structures and articular involvement (5,8,20).

Besides demonstration of vascular involvement and the relationship of
tumor to adjacent blood vessels, ANGIOGRAPHY is of little or no value in
the evaluation of tumor extent.

1.3 MAGNETIC RESONANCE IMAGING:

On MRI, basic information is comprised in SI of various tissues, which is
determined by various parameters (proton density, relaxation times, flow
phenomena,...) and by selection of different pulse sequences. This
multiplicity of parameters is responsible for the extremely high contrast
resolution of the method. A summary of these parameters, as well as the
MRI-appearance of normal musculoskeletal structures, is presented in
section 1.4.

Neoplastic tissues have an increased amount of extra- and intracellular free
water and consequently have longer T1 and T2 relaxation times. Moreover,
the T1 relaxation time appears to be correlated with the rate of cell division
and the phase of mitosis, even when the total amount of cell water is
constant. These biophysical phenomena make proton MRI a potentially
valuable method in tumor diagnosis and staging (10).

By combining outstanding contrast resolution and high spatial resolution,
MRI offers a tremendous potential for the *detection, diagnosis* and *staging*
of musculoskeletal neoplasms. This explains an increased use of MRI for
the investigation of bone and soft tissue tumors during the past three years.

However, because of the excellence of conventional methods, long
MR-examination time, poor availability of MR-installations and economic
considerations, at the present time, MRI is not suitable for screening
purposes (i.e. lesion *detection*).

Diagnosis is based on morphological information by changed SI and on
the SI itself, allowing more specific histological characterization.

Finally, high contrast resolution combined with the multiplanar imaging
ability (to directly obtain images in nearly any desired plane) are responsible
for the accurate *staging* capability, i.e. evaluation of extent, by MRI.

Increased morphological information by MRI allows a more accurate
classification of the local behaviour of musculoskeletal neoplasms compared
to the CR-classification, mentioned in table 1.1. A summary of the
morphological MRI-characteristics, allowing differentiation between
non-aggressive (usually benign) and aggressive (usually malignant) tumors
is presented in table 1.2 (3,12,13,22).

Table 1.2: Morphological MRI-criteria for non-aggressive (benign) and aggressive
(malignant) tumors:

Benign:	Malignant:
homogeneous	inhomogeneous (irregular, poorly defined)
sharp margins (low signal rim between tumor and marrow)	indistinct margins ('dirty cortex') infiltration of the surrounding fat involvement of more than one muscle group or compartment thickening of the surrounding muscles increased T2-SI of the surrounding muscles

Considering the same morphological information by MRI-SI and the SI itself,
MRI is the method of choice for differentiation between normal structures
and pathological conditions.
Hence, MRI also easily differentiates between normal structures like marrow
(fat), bone, muscle, fibrocartilage, ligaments, tendons, nerves, blood vessels
and pathologic conditions like fluid collections (cysts, liquefaction, necrosis,
fluid-fluid levels), increased tissue water content (tumor, edema,
inflammation), hemorrhage, ectopic bone or fat, and fibrous tissue.

Cortical bone generates no signal due to the lack of mobile protons. Nevertheless, ossification, calcification and periosteal new bone formation can be recognized by their signal void, which on the contrary lacks specificity as it may also be caused by flowing blood, fibrous tissue or air. Cortical bone involvement can be roughly demonstrated by changes in configuration (mottled appearance) and by raise in signal intensity on T2-weighted images (grey instead of black). CR and CT, however, remain the methods of choice in demonstrating cortical bone pathology and ectopic calcification or ossification.

Bone marrow generates a high signal on MRI because of the presence of abundant fat. Exception made for calcification or ossification, medullary involvement, i.e. replacement of fat by tumoral tissue, results in decreased SI on T1-weighted images and increased SI on T2-weighted images. Based on this pronounced changes of SI of bone marrow when involved, accurate assessment of intramedullary tumor extent is possible, as illustrated in Fig. 1.3.

Soft tissue invasion causes an increased SI being always higher than that of involved marrow.
According to Zimmer, tumor detection with MRI is based on these three phenomena (cortical, medullary and/or soft tissue invasion)(22).

The relative SI of musculoskeletal tissues and fluids, occurring in normal and pathologic conditions on both most commonly used spin echo sequences are summarized in table 1.3. (2,4,6,10,12).

Table 1.3: Spectrum of SI of normal musculoskeletal structures and in major pathologic conditions:

T1-weighted images:	T2-weighted images:
Highest signal intensity	
(Short T1-relaxation time)	(Long T2-relaxation time)
Fat (adipose tissue, bone marrow)	Free water Stagnant blood Proteinaceous fluid
Subacute, chronic hemorrhage (> 7 days)	Fresh hemorrhage (< 1 day) Subacute, chronic hemorrhage (> 7 days)
Hyaline cartilage	Fat
Nonneoplastic tumor tissue	Hyaline cartilage
Muscle	Muscle
Fibrocartilage	Acute hemorrhage (1-6 days)
Proteinaceous fluid (synovial fluid)	
Free water (edema, stagnant blood, neoplastic tissue, cyst fluid, necrosis, intervertebral disk)	
Fresh (< 1 day) and acute hemorrhage (1-6 days)	
Ligaments and tendons	Ligaments and tendons
Scars (also hemosiderin in post-hemorrhagic scars)	Scars (posthemorrhagic scars)
Cortical bone	Cortical bone
Air	Air
(Long T1-relaxation time)	(Short T2-relaxation time)
Lowest Signal intensity	

Based on this classification, MR-image interpretation will have optimal tissue characterizing abilities (10).
Tissue characterization only by means of the calculation of relaxation times, however, is found less reliable because of significant overlapping, large variations in different tumor components and poor reproducibility (3).

The ultimate goal is to find specific MRI-characteristics for definite tumors and tumor components. This may be possible by combining SI of the lesion with its morphological appearance, as illustrated for various tumor components in a case of liposarcoma (Fig. 1.4).
Likewise, MR-criteria have been described for various bone and soft tissue tumors as discussed in the corresponding chapters.

Adequate staging of musculoskeletal neoplasms is not only important if surgery is considered, but also facilitates radiation therapy planning (15). Furthermore, response to conservative treatment can be evaluated by changes in signal intensity (1,22).
Detection of residual or recurrent tumor after surgery and/or radiation therapy is based on the ability of MRI to differentiate between fibrous and non fibrous tissue (11,19). Increased SI after non-surgical therapy may be due either to a remaining or recurrent active tumor, or to intratumoral necrosis and edema, indicating a good response to therapy (20).
The use of intravenous paramagnetic contrast media (mainly shortening the T1 relaxation time) further improves the already excellent contrast resolution of MRI (17) and, as discussed below, may enable a more specific diagnosis.

Although important, considerations such as high cost and a long duration of the MRI-examination — representing the main disadvantages of MRI -, as well as its complete non-invasive nature — being a major advantage — are beyond the scope of its value in the assessment of bone and soft tissue neoplasms and, therefore, will not be discussed furthermore.

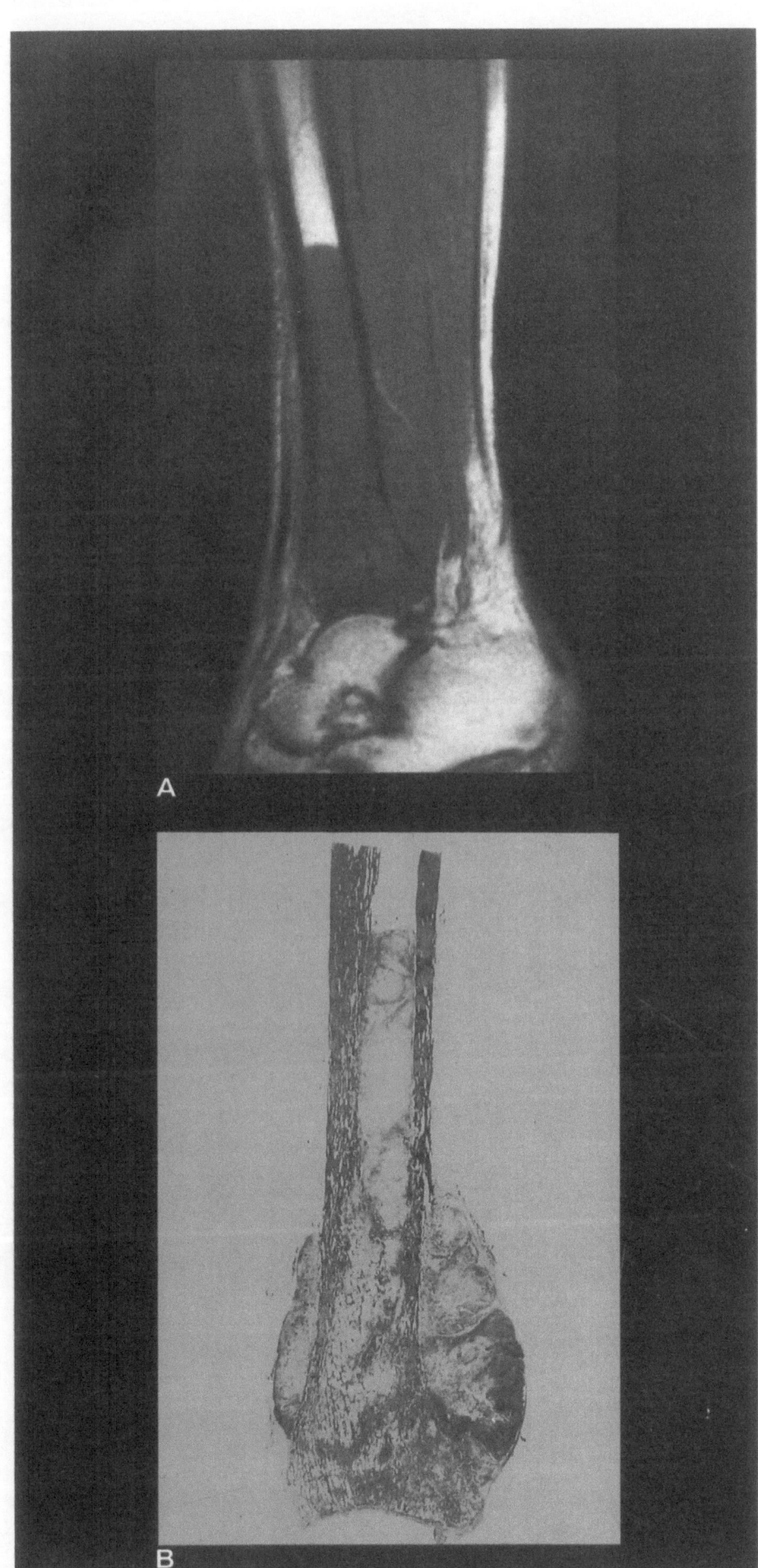

Fig. 1.3. G.H., 44 year-old male.

1.3.a. MRI of the left tibia and ankle,
sagittal section, T1-WI.
Replacement of medullary fat by low
SI [3] tumor tissue at the distal part
of the tibia. Sharp and small transition
at the cranial border. Increased SI of
the uninvolved marrow may be
explained by the 'pushing '
phenomenon. Extension into the
paraosseous soft tissues anteriorly
and posteriorly to the distal metaphysis
of the tibia.

1.3.b. Macroscopic specimen. (Courtesy
Prof Van Damme,KUL)
Replacement of the medullary fat by
abnormal tissue, which is sharply
demarcated at the top. Paraosseous
involvement at the distal part, both
anteriorly and posteriorly to the tibia.

Diagnosis: Chondrosarcoma.
The remarkable similarity between
MRI- and pathologic findings, illustrating
the accurate staging capability by
MRI, is shown.

14

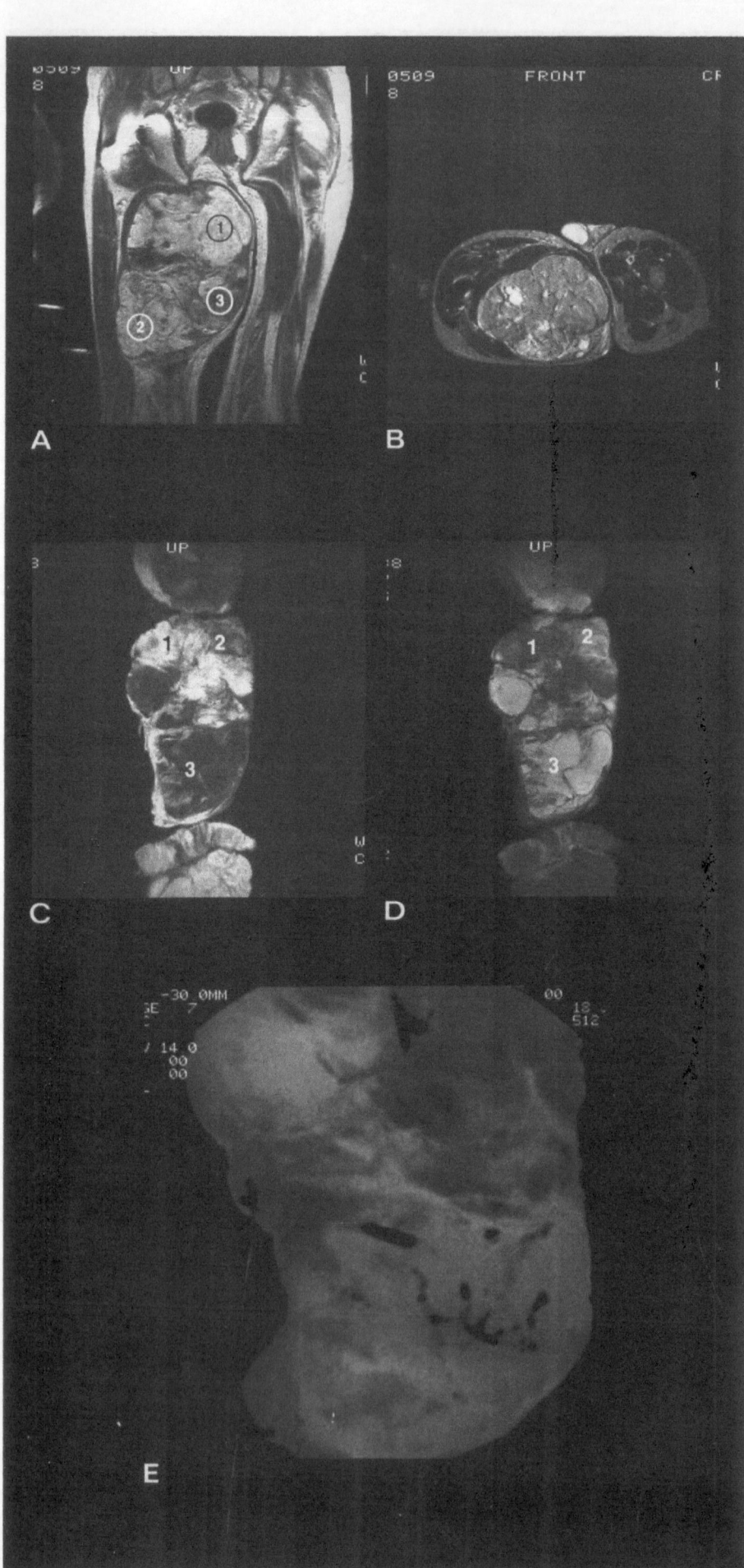

Fig. 1.4. D.V.J., 48 year-old male.

1.4.a. MRI of the thigh, coronal section, T1-WI.

  Large polylobulated soft tissue mass in the right thigh. Tumor lobules have a variable SI from extremely high [8] (area 1) over intermediate [4] (area 2) to very low [2] (area 3).

1.4.b. MRI of the thigh region, transverse section, T2-WI.

  As the level is at the cranial part of the tumor (area 1 in Fig.1.4.a), only lobules with high and extremely high SI [6] [8] are demonstrated.

1.4.c and d. MRI of the resected specimen, T1-WI (c) and T2-WI (d).

  The same areas of different SI, as mentioned in Fig. 1.4.a, are demonstrated again.

1.4.e. CT of the resected specimen.

  Contrast between the various areas, mentioned in Fig. 1.4.a, is also seen, but is less obvious than on MRI.

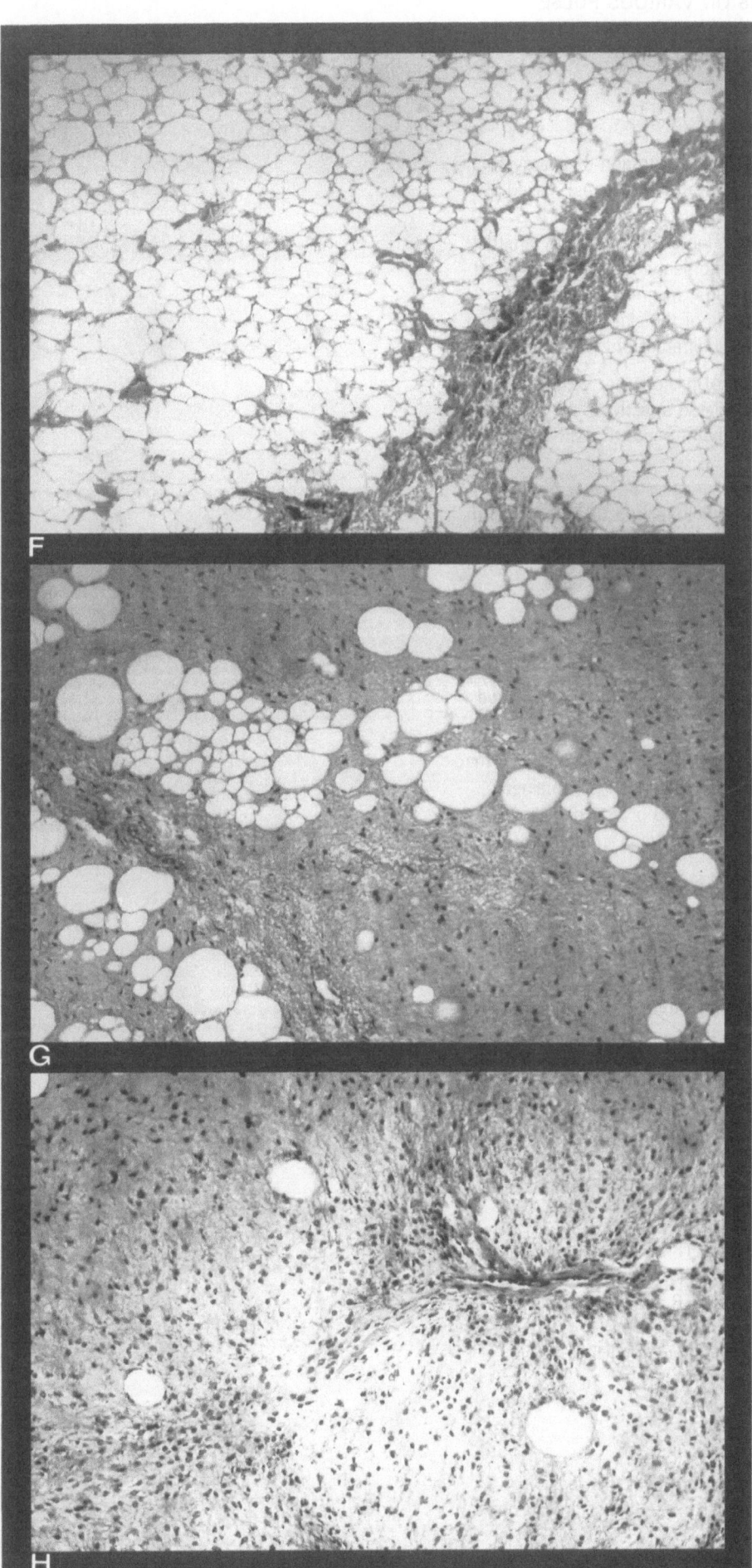

1.4.f, g and h. Microphotographs of the
resected specimen.
  f. Well differentiated part with
  preponderance of fat cells (lipomatous
  component).
  g. Moderate amount of irregular fat
  cells and presence of myxoid tissue
  (myxoid component).
  h. Myxoid tissue without fat cells
  (sarcomatous component).
Diagnosis: Liposarcoma.
  This case illustrates the tissue
  characterizing capabilities of MRI,
  based on SI.

16

1.4 FUNDAMENTALS OF MRI – MRI-APPEARANCE OF NORMAL MUSCULOSKELETAL STRUCTURES ON VARIOUS PULSE SEQUENCES (T1-,T2- and PROTON DENSITY SPIN-ECHO and STIR IMAGES).

1.4.1. Fundamentals of MRI:

Basically, magnetic resonance consists of an administration of energy to protons within a selected plane (under the form of radiowaves), called the radiofrequency pulse (*RF-pulse*), followed by delivery of the absorbed energy by these protons. The latter phenomenon also happens by emitting radiowaves ('the MR-signal'). The whole phenomenon is called resonance, and since it happens in a strong magnetic field: 'magnetic resonance'. The strength of this MR-signal forms the basis of the signal intensity on MR-images and is mainly determined by three different physical parameters:

1/ PROTON DENSITY, reflecting the number of protons per volume unit. As a rule, strength of emitted MR-signal is related directly to the proton density: the more protons per volume unit, the stronger the MR-signal, and hence the higher SI.
2/ T1-RELAXATION TIME, being a parameter for the facility of delivery of absorbed energy. On SE-images, SI is inversely related to T1-relaxation time: the longer T1, the lower SI and vice versa.
3/ T2-RELAXATION TIME, which is a parameter for the homogeneity of the magnetic field at the level of the protons in a tissue, and influenced by the chemical composition of that tissue. On SE-images SI is related directly to T2-relaxation time: the longer T2, the higher SI and vice versa. For a detailed description of these parameters, as for an extensive description of MR-physics, we refer to excellent books and articles, listed below (16,21).

With spin echo sequences, as used in nearly all MR-examinations performed in the cases presented below, three groups of images can be obtained, by varying pulse sequence parameters: T1-, T2- and proton density weighted images.

Although already mentioned, it is important to stress that *for all MR-images SI is determined by the influence of T1, T2 and proton density at the same time*. However, the influence of one of these parameters can be enhanced, by using an appropriate pulse sequence, resulting in T1-, T2- or proton density weighted images. This is illustrated in Fig. 1.5 a to c, representing images with different weighting of a transverse section at the same level of the knee region.
For comparison, four test tubes with different content are placed behind the knee and also imaged. The tube in the centre of the image (left tube, indicated with "B") (tube 1) is filled with fresh, unclotted blood; the second tube (also "B",tube 2) contains serum of clotted blood; tube 3 (indicated with " W") contains water; the tube most at the right side of the image (tube 4), indicated with "F", is filled with a fatty substance.

Summarized, for spin echo sequences,
– a T1-weighted image is obtained when both TR and TE are short (i.e. TR < 0.7 sec and TE < 40 msec at 0.5 T);
– a T2-weighted image is obtained when both TR and TE are long (i.e. TR > 1.5 sec and TE > 60 msec at 0.5 T);
– a proton density image is obtained when TR is long while TE is short (i.e. TR > 1.5 sec and TE < 40 msec at 0.5 T)

1.4.2 T1-weighted image (Fig.1.5.a):

As a rule, on T1-weighted images, SI is correlated with the density of protons and inversely with T1-relaxation time (i.e. the higher proton density, the higher SI; the longer T1, the lower SI).
For example: fat has a high proton density and a very short T1 and hence appears very bright on T1-WI; synovial fluid, although it has a relatively

high proton density, appears dark because of its very long T1; cortical bone appears dark by lack of mobile protons.

On the T1-weighted image of the knee, the spectrum of SI is as follows (see also table 1.3 in this chapter) (Fig.1.5.a):

high SI:	fatty tissue (subcutaneous fat — bone marrow)
	hyaline cartilage (articular surface)
	muscle
	synovial fluid (seen as a curvilinear, low intensity area anterolaterally of the lateral condyle of the femur)
	menisci
	ligaments — tendons — joint capsule
	cortical bone
low SI:	streaming blood

As demonstrated, on T1-WI, fat tissue is particularly well shown. Therefore, with respect to bone tumors, the contrast between tumor and fat (including bone marrow and subcutaneous fat) is improved on these images.

1.4.3 proton density-weighted image (Fig.1.5.b):

As a rule, on proton density-weighted images, SI mainly depends on density of protons (i.e. the higher proton density, the higher SI).

On the proton density-weighted image of the knee, the following spectrum of SI is noted (Fig.1.5.b):

high SI:	fatty tissue
	hyaline cartilage
	synovial fluid
	muscle
	menisci
	ligaments — tendons — joint capsule
	cortical bone
low SI:	streaming blood

1.4.4 T2-weighted image (Figure 1.5.c):

As a rule, on T2-weighted images, SI is correlated with both density of protons and T2-relaxation time (i.e. the higher proton density, the higher SI; the longer T2, the higher SI).
For example: joint fluid has a high proton density and a very long T2 and hence appears very bright on T2-WI; fat has also a high proton density and a long T2 and has therefore also a high SI; muscle has a high proton density, but only an intermediate T2 and thus appears of intermediate SI.

On the T2-WI image of the knee, the following spectrum of SI is observed (see also table 1.3 in this chapter) (Fig.1.5.c):

high SI:	synovial fluid
	stagnant blood (see test tube 1 and 2)
	fatty tissue
	hyaline cartilage
	muscle
	cortical bone
low SI:	streaming blood

As in tumor T2 is markedly prolongated, causing high SI on T2-WI, while muscle has a low SI, it is easily understood that the differentiation between tumor and muscle is most obvious on T2-WI.

1.4.5 Short-T1-inversion-recovery (STIR):

STIR is another pulse sequence, that mainly provides T1-contrast in the images. As it was only sparsely applicated in our series, this sequence will not be discussed in detail.

Essentially, as mentioned before, differences in T1 are enhanced when using this sequence, i.e. tissues with short T1 will appear bright on STIR-images, whereas tissues or structures with even a slight prolongation of T1 will appear much more darker, the contrast being more pronounced than on corresponding T1-weighted spin-echo-images.

As a result, with respect to the material discussed, STIR-images are very useful in exact determining intraosseous extent of bone tumors.

In fig. 1.5.d. a transverse STIR-image, at the same level as in figures 1.5.a-c. is presented. As can be observed, structures and tissues with prolongated T1, such as joint fluid, stagnant blood (test tubes 1 and 2) and muscle contrast very well with others, having a short T1 (like fat).

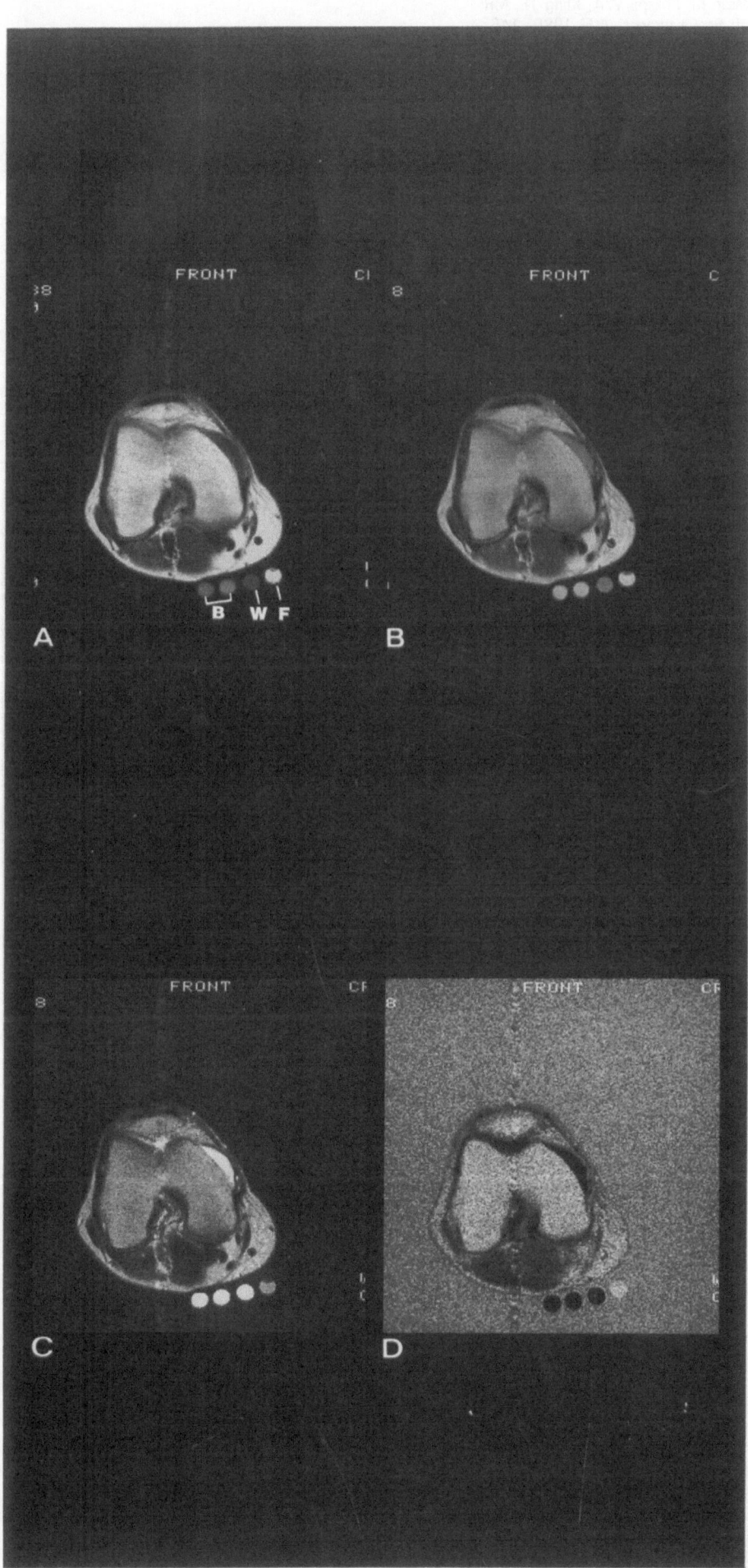

Fig. 1.5. MRI, transverse sections at the same level of the knee in a normal individual.

a. Spin echo sequence, T1-weighted image (TR: 0.5 sec, TE: 30 msec)
b. Spin echo sequence, Proton density weighted image (TR: 1.6 sec, TE: 30 msec)
c. Spin echo sequence, T2-weighted image (TR: 1,6 sec, TE: 90 msec)
d. STIR-sequence, T1-image (TR: 1.8 sec, TE: 35 msec, TI: 140 msec)

Legends are described in the text.

20

References

1. Aisen AM, Martel W, Braunstein EM, McMillin KI, Phillips WA, Kling TF. MRI and CT evaluation of primary bone and soft tissue tumors. AJR 1986; 146: 749-756.
2. Baleriaux D., Coussement A. Voyage au pays des protons. Editions Vigot, 1988, Paris.
3. Beltran J, Simon DC, Katz W, Weis LD. Increased MR signal intensity in skeletal muscle adjacent to malignant tumors: pathologic correlation and clinical relevance. Radiology 1987; 162: 251-255.
4. Bloem JL, Bluemm RG, Taminiau AHM, van Oosterom AT, Stolk J, Doornbos J. Magnetic resonance imaging of primary malignant bone tumors. RadioGraphics 1987; 7(3): 425-445.
5. Demas BE, Heelan RT, Lane J, Marcove R, Hajdu S, Brennan MF. Soft-tissue sarcomas of the extremities: comparison of MR and CT in determining the extent of disease. AJR 1988; 150: 615-620.
6. Dooms GC, Fisher MR, Hricak H, Richardson M, Crooks LE, Genant HK. Bone marrow imaging: magnetic resonance studies related to age and sex. Radiology 1985; 155: 429-432.
7. Freiberger R. Thougts on the diagnosis of bone tumors. Radiology 1984; 150: 276.
8. Gillespy III Th., Manfrini M., Ruggieri P. et al. Staging of intraosseous extent of osteosarcoma: correlation of preoperative CT and MR imaging with pathologic macroslides. Radiology 1988; 167: 765-767
9. Lodwick GS. Atlas of tumor radiology. The bones and joints. Year Book Medical Publishers 1971, Chicago.
10. Mitchell DG, Burk DL, Vinitski S, Rifkin MD. The biophysical basis of tissue contrast in extracranial MR imaging. AJR 1987; 149: 831-837.
11. Moon KL, Genant HK, Helms CA, Chafetz NI, Crooks LE, Kaufman L. Musculoskeletal applications of nuclear magnetic resonance. Radiology 1983; 147: 161-171.
12. Murphy WA, Totty WG. Musculoskeletal magnetic resonance imaging. Magnetic Resonance Annual 1986. edited by Herbert Y. Kressel. Raven Press, New York.
13. Petasnick JP, Turner DA, Charters JR, Gitelis S, Zacharias CE. Soft-tissue masses of the locomotor system: comparison of MR imaging with CT. Radiology 1986; 160: 125-133.
14. Petterson H, Springfield DS, Enneking WF. Radiological management of musculoskeletal tumors. Springer-Verlag. London Berlin Heidelberg New York Paris Tokio, 1987.
15. Porter BA. MR may become routine for imaging bone marrow. Diagn Imaging 1987; : 104-108.
16. Pykett IL, Newhouse JH, Brady TJ. Principles of nuclear magnetic resonance imaging. Radiology 1982; 143: 157-168
17. Richardson ML, Kilcoyne RF, Gillespy III T, Helms CA, Genant HK. Magnetic resonance imaging of musculoskeletal neoplasms. Radiol Clin North Am 1986; 24(2): 259-267.
18. Totty WG, Murphy WA, Lee JKT. Soft-tissue tumors: MR imaging. Radiology 1986; 160: 135-141.
19. Vanel D, Lacombe MJ, Couanet D, Kalifa C, Spielmann M, Genin J. Musculoskeletal tumors: follow-up with MR imaging after treatment with surgery and radiation therapy. Radiology 1987; 164: 243-245.
20. Wetzel LH, Levine E, Murphey MD. A comparison of MR imaging and CT in the evaluation of musculoskeletal masses. RadioGraphics 1987; 7(5): 851-874.
21. Young SW: Nuclear magnetic resonance imaging, basic principles. Raven Press 1984: 11-91.
22. Zimmer WD, Berquiot TH, MoLood RA, Sim FH et al. Bone tumors: magnetic resonance imaging versus computed tomography. Radiology 1985; 155: 709-718.

CHAPTER 2

MATERIALS AND METHODS:

During a period of 17 months (from 01.01.1987 until 30.05.1988) 275
new cases of bone and soft tissue tumors in the province of Antwerp
(1 200 000 inhabitants) have been registrated.
With the cooperation of the referring clinicians 94 cases were investigated
by magnetic resonance imaging.
For reasons of differential diagnosis some non-neoplastic, non-tumoral
lesions (like osteomyelitis, fibrous dysplasia, Paget's disease, stress fracture,
bone infarction) were also examined by MRI. Evident cases of metastatic
disease were excluded. Except for vertebral hemangiomas, only patients
with histologically proven diagnosis from either surgical or biopsy specimens
are included in this study. Finally, 88 cases were retained (Table 2.1).

Table 2.1: Histologic groups of lesions studied (n = 88).

Lesions	No.
Benign bone tumors	
osteoid osteoma	7
enchondroma	2
DD bone infarct	2
osteochondroma	5
giant cell tumor	4
vertebral hemangioma	6
solitary bone cyst	4
aneurysmal bone cyst	3
non ossifying fibroma	2
eosinophilic granuloma	2
DD fibrous dysplasia	6
DD Paget's disease	1
DD osteomyelitis	3
Malignant bone tumors	
osteogenic sarcoma	10
DD stress fracture	3
chondrosarcoma	4
myeloma	2
metastatic disease	6
Benign soft tissue tumors	
lipoma	2
schwannoma	1
neurofibroma	2
soft tissue hemangioma	1
aggressive fibromatosis	1
(myositis ossificans	1)
Malignant soft tissue tumors	
liposarcoma	4
malignant fibrous histiocytoma	2
rhabdomyosarcoma	2

The purposes of the study were:
1. determination of the value of MRI for the diagnosis and staging in a
statistically significant series of bone and soft tissue neoplasms.
2. comparison of the value of MRI with that of the other available imaging
modalities (scintigraphy, conventional radiography, CT, angiography and
DSA) both for diagnosis and for staging of these tumors.
3. determination of the value of the use of paramagnetic contrast agents
(Gadolinium-DTPA) for diagnostic and staging purposes in a series of 32
patients.

MRI-images were obtained using a 1.0 T superconductive magnet, operating at .5 T (Magnetom, Siemens AG).

Multisection spin echo techniques were commonly used, with slice thickness of 5 to 7 mm and intersection gap of 0 to 7 mm, depending on the size of the lesion and that of the involved bone.

When located in the trunk, the standard body coil was used. In cases of location in the extremities, the study was performed using the standard head coil or Helmholtz coil. Lesions of the spine were examined with the spine surface coil.

In all cases proton density-, T1- and T2-weighted images were obtained in a different spatial plane (most commonly coronal T1 and transverse proton density and T2).

Short T1- inversion recovery sequences (STIR) were used rather exceptionally and may allow a better visualization of marrow pathology.

As paramagnetic contrast agents mainly influence T1-relaxation time, only T1-weighted sequences were repeated after intravenous injection of Gd-DTPA (Schering AG). Prior to this administration of Gd-DTPA, informed consent was obtained in all cases, corresponding to the recommendations of the Ethic Committee of the University Hospital of Antwerp.
Gd-DTPA was administrated intravenously in a dose of 0.2 ml/kg weight.

Both on T1- and T2-weighted images signal intensities of all lesions were semiquantitatively determined. For uniform lesions (f.i. uniform giant cell tumor) SI was determined all over the tumor, whereas in cases of complex lesions, this was done for all tumor components (f.i. in osteoid osteoma in the region of hyperostosis, of the nidus and of the central calcification). The signal intensity of the lesion was compared to that of normal subcutaneous fat and muscle both on T1- and T2- weighted images.
In the subsequent so-called spin-echo greyscale, SI of the lesions vary from [0] up to [8]: [0] means absence of signal (f.i.cortical bone), [3]: SI equal to that of muscle, [6]: SI of fat and [8]: much brighter than fat, on T2-WI corresponding to the SI of free water (Table 2.2). Throughout all presented cases, numbers between brackets [] refer to this scale.

Table 2.2 MR-grey scale

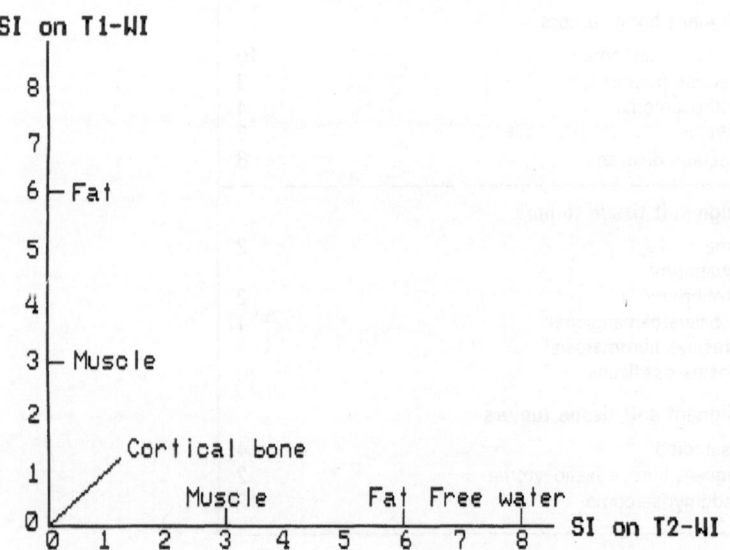

Similar lesions are grouped and their MRI-characteristics will be discussed and compared with literature data. The SE-grey scale will be completed with more specific data characteristic for various tumors and tumor components and is displayed at the end of each chapter, when at least three cases were available.

The reproducable value of this SE-grey scale, the relative utility of different imaging modalities and the results of the contrast study will be the basis for the general conclusions.

BENIGN BONE TUMORS
AND MIMICKING CONDITIONS

CHAPTER 3

OSTEOID OSTEOMA

Osteoid osteoma represents 10 to 12% of all benign bone tumors. Patients are frequently young adults, consulting with a history of intermittent or continuous pain occurring mostly at night and which is relieved by salicylates. Femur, tibia, hands and feet are the most frequent locations. Histologically it consists of a central area (nidus) of highly vascularized osteoblastic connective tissue and osteoid (bone resembling substance), often containing varying amounts of calcification and surrounded by a zone of reactive hyperostotic bone (4).

CR and CT-characteristics have been well described (1). Central hypolucent nidus with or without calcification and surrounding hyperdense bone gives the entire lesion a "bull's-eye" appearance.

MR-literature is very sparse.
Glass described the MR-features of the lesion as a low SI-ring (calcification) surrounded by an irregular area of high SI (nidus) and a rim of low SI (hyperostosis) (2).
Widening of the neighbouring joint by material of high SI on T2-WI is thought to represent synovial thickening or fluid. There is increased SI of the surrounding bone marrow on T2-WI, most likely due to an inflammatory response.
No contrast studies are described in the literature.
According to Wetzel (5) osteoid osteoma is better evaluated by CT compared to MR!

References

1. Gamba JL, Martinez S, Apple J, Harrelson JM, Nunley JA. Computed tomography of axial skeletal osteoid osteomas. AJR 1984; 142: 769-772.
2. Glass RBJ, Poznanski AK, Fisher MR, Shkolnik A, Dias L. MR imaging of osteoid osteoma. J Comput Assist Tomogr 1986; 10(6): 1065-1067.
3. Helms CA, Hattner RS, Vogler III JB. Osteoid osteoma: radionuclide diagnosis. Radiology 1984;151:779-784.
4. Van Rompaey W, Vereycken H, De Schepper A. Diagnosis of osteoid osteoma by digital subtraction angiography. Fortschr Röntgenstr 1986; 145(5): 578-581.
5. Wetzel LH, Levine E, Murphey MD. A comparison of MR imaging and CT in the evaluation of musculoskeletal masses. RadioGraphics 1987; 7(5): 851-874.

26

COMMENT

1. Morphological evaluation of osteoid osteomas by MRI is based on the same basic signs as it is on CR and CT ("bull's eye").

2. Our series comprises seven patients with osteoid osteoma. The nidus was seen in all seven cases as a ringlike or rounded area of intermediate SI on T1-WI and of relatively high SI on T2-WI. Central calcification of the nidus, present in four cases, and peripheral hyperostosis in all cases were seen as areas generating no signal on both SE-sequences. Surrounding medullary involvement had an intermediate SI on T1-WI and a relatively high SI on T2-WI and was seen in three cases. Synovial thickening or fluid at the adjacent joints was seen only once.

3. Two of our cases were studied after intravenous injection of Gd-DTPA. There was no definite enhancement of the nidus. Central calcification and reactive hyperostosis remained identical while surrounding marrow involvement became less obvious after contrast injection.

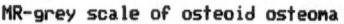

MR-grey scale of osteoid osteoma

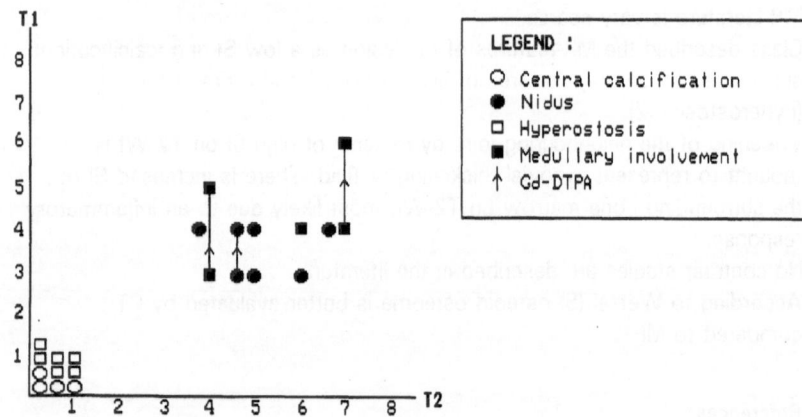

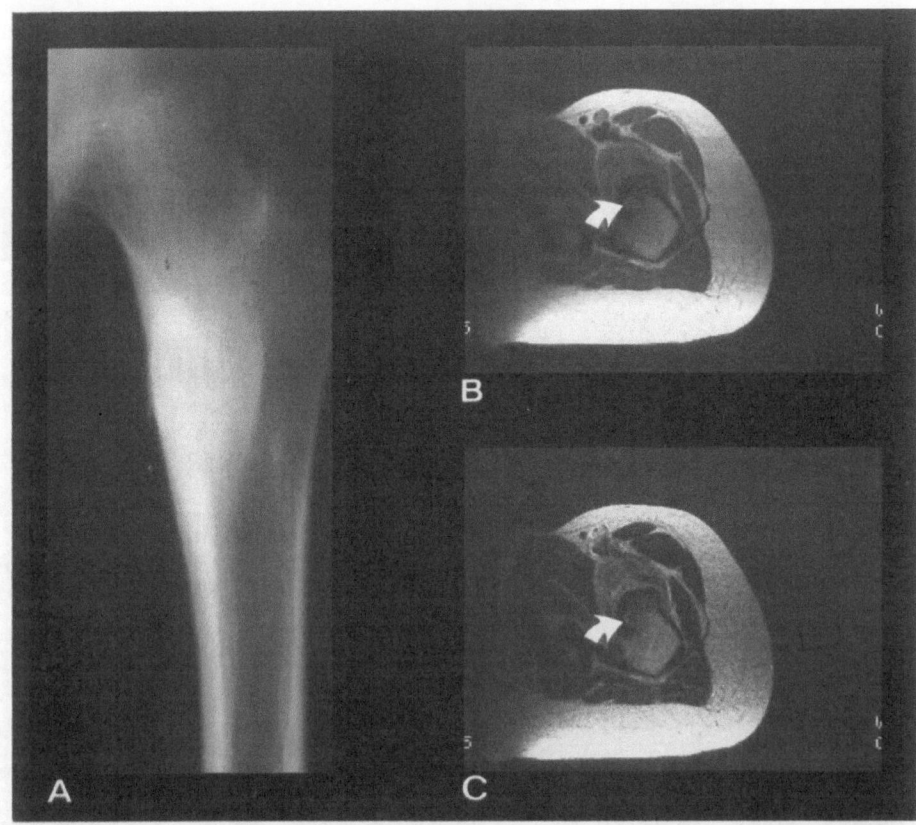

Fig. 3.1. S.P., 11 year-old female.

3.1.a. CR of the left femur.
Ill defined area of hyperostosis at the
left lesser trochanteric region with
central hyperlucency.

3.1.b and c. MRI of the left femur,
transverse section. Proton density-image
(b) and T2-WI (c).
On both images the nidus has a high
SI [6](curved arrow). The central
calcification and the reactive
hyperostosis have a low SI [1].

Diagnosis: Osteoid osteoma.

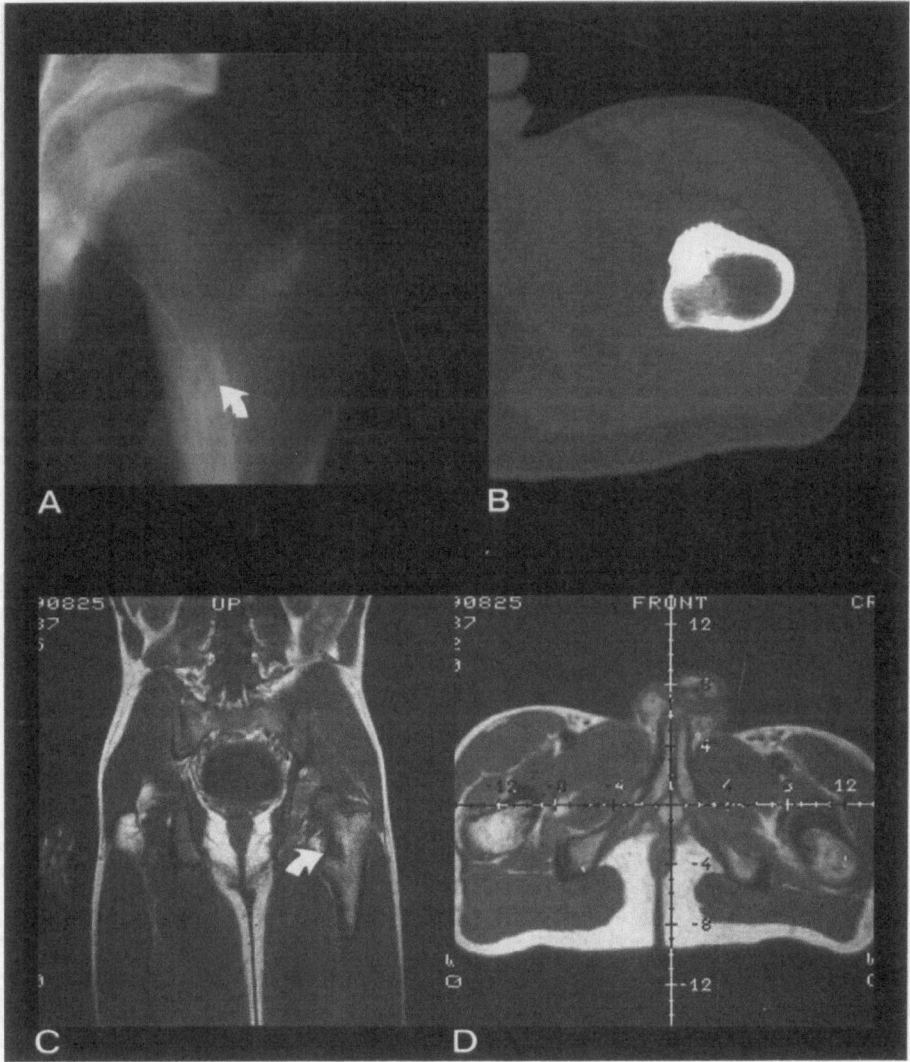

Fig. 3.2. L.K., 17 year-old male.

3.2.a. CR of the left femur.
Ill defined area of hyperostosis craniad
to the lesser trochanter. Central
calcification surrounded by a hypolucent
halo (curved arrow).

3.2.b. CT of the left femur, bone window.
The same findings as on CR are
confirmed.

3.2.c. MRI of the left femur, coronal
section T1-WI.
At this level the nidus is seen as an
area of intermediate SI, surrounded
by a small ring of low SI (curved arrow).

3.2.d. MRI of the left femur, transverse
section, proton density-image.
All three components of the lesion
are demonstrated again.

Diagnosis: Osteoid osteoma

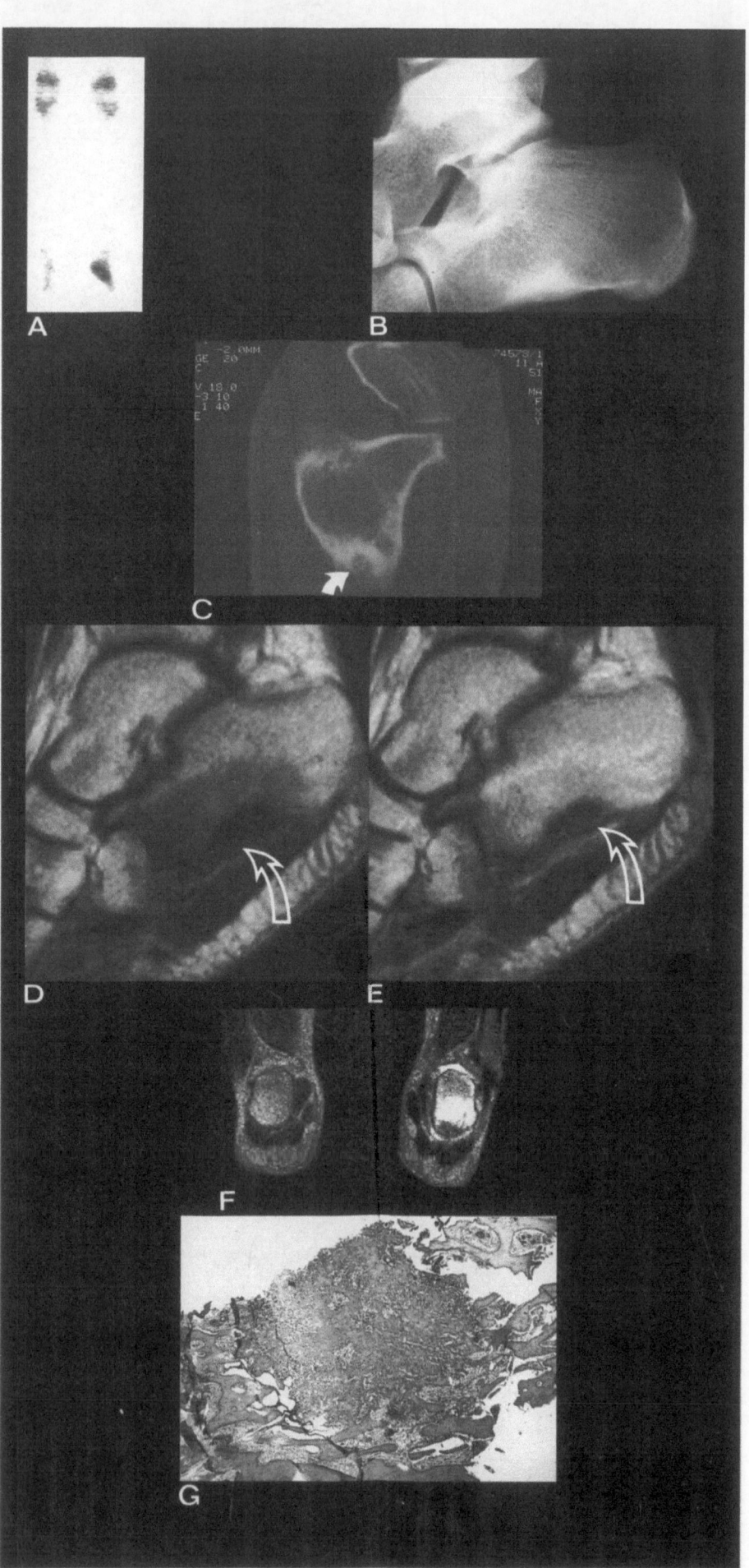

Fig. 3.3. D.L.A., 17 year-old female.

3.3.a. RNSC of the lower legs.
Localized tracer hyperfixation with
central defect at the left heel. The
extent of the hyperfixation is definitely
greater than the extent of the lesion
on conventional radiography.

3.3.b. CR of the right heel.
Crescent shaped zone of hyperostosis
at the plantar side of the left calcaneum.
The lesion appears relatively
homogeneous and has ill defined
margins. There is no cortical destruction.
A localized periosteal reaction is noted.
Adjacent soft tissue appears normal.

3.3.c. CT of the right heel, oblique section,
bone window.
The localized hyperostosis, the unsharp
inner margins and the periosteal
reaction are confirmed. In addition a
tiny calcified fleck can be seen within
a central hypolucent zone (curved
arrow).

3.3.d. MRI of the right heel, sagittal
section, T1-WI.
Within the area of hyperostosis,
generating no signal, a ringlike structure
of higher SI is seen (open curved
arrow). The area of hyperostosis is
surrounded by a medullary zone of
intermediate SI.

3.3.e. MRI of the right heel, sagittal section,
T1-WI after intravenous injection of
Gd-DTPA.
Preferential enhancement of the
surrounding medullary zone. In
comparison to fig. 3.3.d. contrast
with normal medulla becomes less
obvious.
Slight enhancement of the nidus
(curved open arrow).

3.3.f. MRI of both heels, coronal section,
T2-WI.
The area of hyperostosis in the right
calcaneum remains of low signal but
is less homogeneous compared to
the T1-WI. The surrounding medullary
zone generates an extremely high
signal. A high signal line is noted both
at the dorsal and the plantar side of
the left calcaneum, due to synovial
thickening or/and fluid and parosteal
inflammation.

3.3.g. Microphotograph, resected specimen.
The nidus is clearly demonstrated
within osteoid material.

Diagnosis: Osteoid osteoma

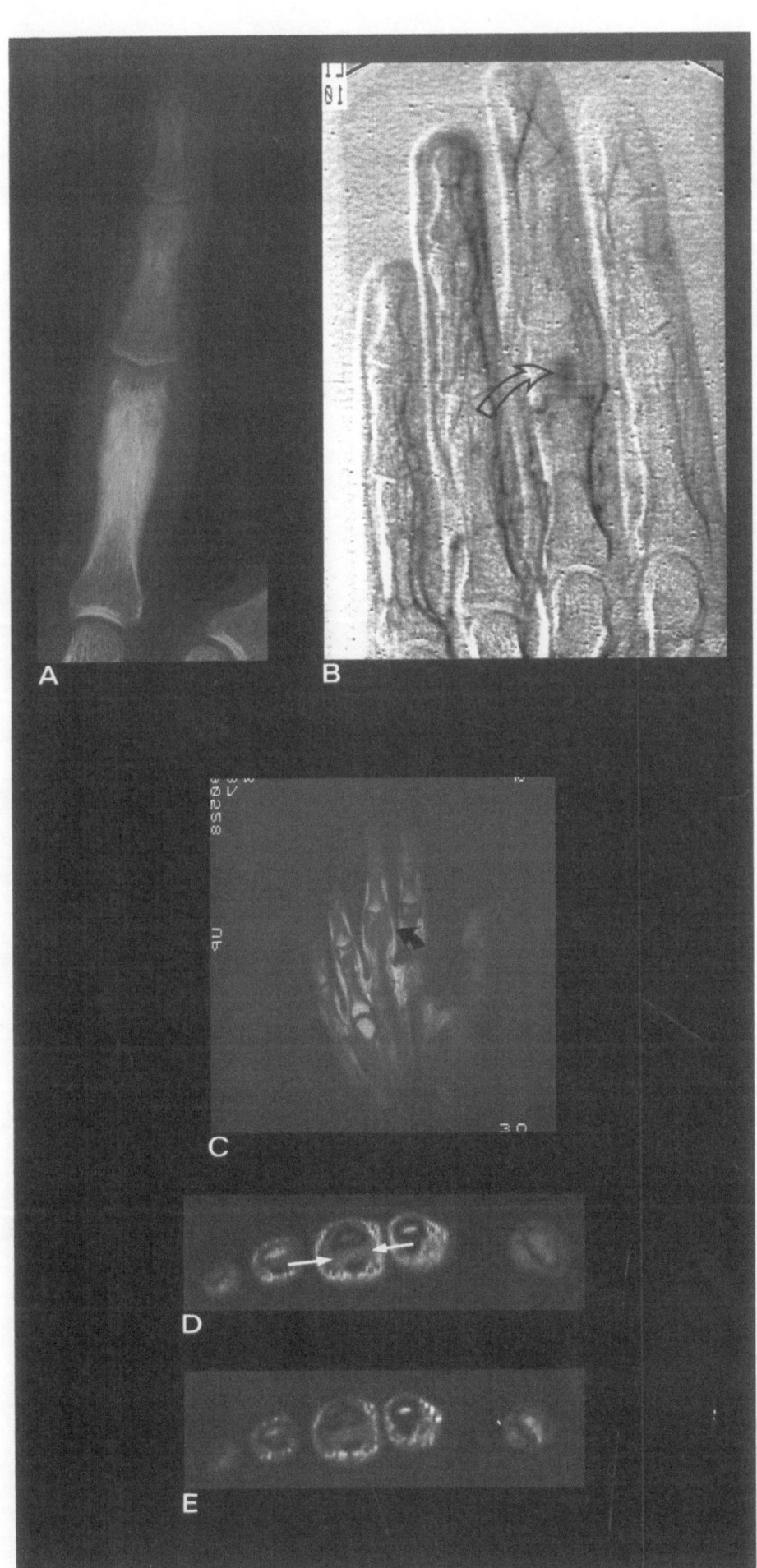

Fig. 3.4. M.C., 18-year-old female.

3.4.a. CR of the left middle finger.
Broadening of the proximal phalanx.
Soft tissue mass.

3.4.b. Intraarterial digital subtraction
angiography of the fingers.
Hypervascular central lesion with
long-standing arteriolar blush. (curved
open arrow).

3.4.c. MRI of the left hand, coronal section,
T1-WI.
Section through the eccentrically
located nidus (curved arrow).
Intermediate SI [3] of the lesion.

3.4.d and e MRI of the left fingers,
transverse section, proton density-(d)
and T2-WI (e).
Relatively high SI of the nidus [5]
(arrows).
Flattened cortical bone with normal SI.
Decreased SI in the medullary cavity [4].

Diagnosis: Osteoid osteoma, confirmed
by core biopsy.

CHAPTER 4

ENCHONDROMA

Enchondroma is a benign cartilage tumor arising within the medullary cavity and originating from cartilage rests displaced from the physis. Hands and feet are most frequently affected.
When arising in long bones the lesion may be symptomatic but usually the lesion is an incidental finding. Age distribution is from the second to the fifth decade. Lesions may be solitary or multiple. Histologically they consist of mature hyaline cartilage interspersed with small uninuclear cartilage cells.
Radiologic examination reveals a radiolucent lesion with cortical expansion and central spotty calcifications. MRI-appearance and configuration of cartilage lesions vary depending on the presence of a hyaline matrix. Enchondromas, containing hyaline cartilage appear as lobules within lobules which are of diffuse high SI on T2-WI (1).

Differential diagnosis: bone infarcts.

Because enchondromas have to be differentiated from bone infarcts, these also are included in our series. Bone infarcts are associated with occlusive vascular disease, hematological disorders, caisson disease, collagen disease, trauma and infection. Femur and tibia are most commonly involved.
Radiologically they present with a serpiginous, densely calcified area in the medullary cavity, and a well defined perilesional sclerosis. Both signs are not seen in enchondroma (2).
MRI-findings of bone infarcts reflect CR-CT-findings and have low SI on both T1- and T2-WI differentiating them from cartilage tumors (2).

References

1. Cohen EK, Kressel HY, Frank TS, Fallon M et al. Hyaline cartilage-origin bone and soft-tissue neoplasms: MR appearance and histologic correlation. Radiology 1988; 167: 477-481.
2. Ehman RL, Berquist TH, McLeod RA. MR imaging of the musculoskeletal system: a 5-year appraisal. Radiology 1988; 166: 313-320.

COMMENT

1. Two cases of enchondroma were evaluated by MRI. Although the first patient presented with characteristic features on CR, MRI-signs of hyaline cartilage as described by Cohen, could not be found (1). We presume that the calcified cartilage matrix, found at biopsy was responsible for the findings on MRI.
In the second case MRI-characteristics as reported by Cohen were confirmed (1).

2. Bone infarcts, although easily recognized on CR-CT, have morphological MRI-characteristics reflecting CR-CT-findings and low SI on both SE-sequences (2).

3. No contrast studies were done.

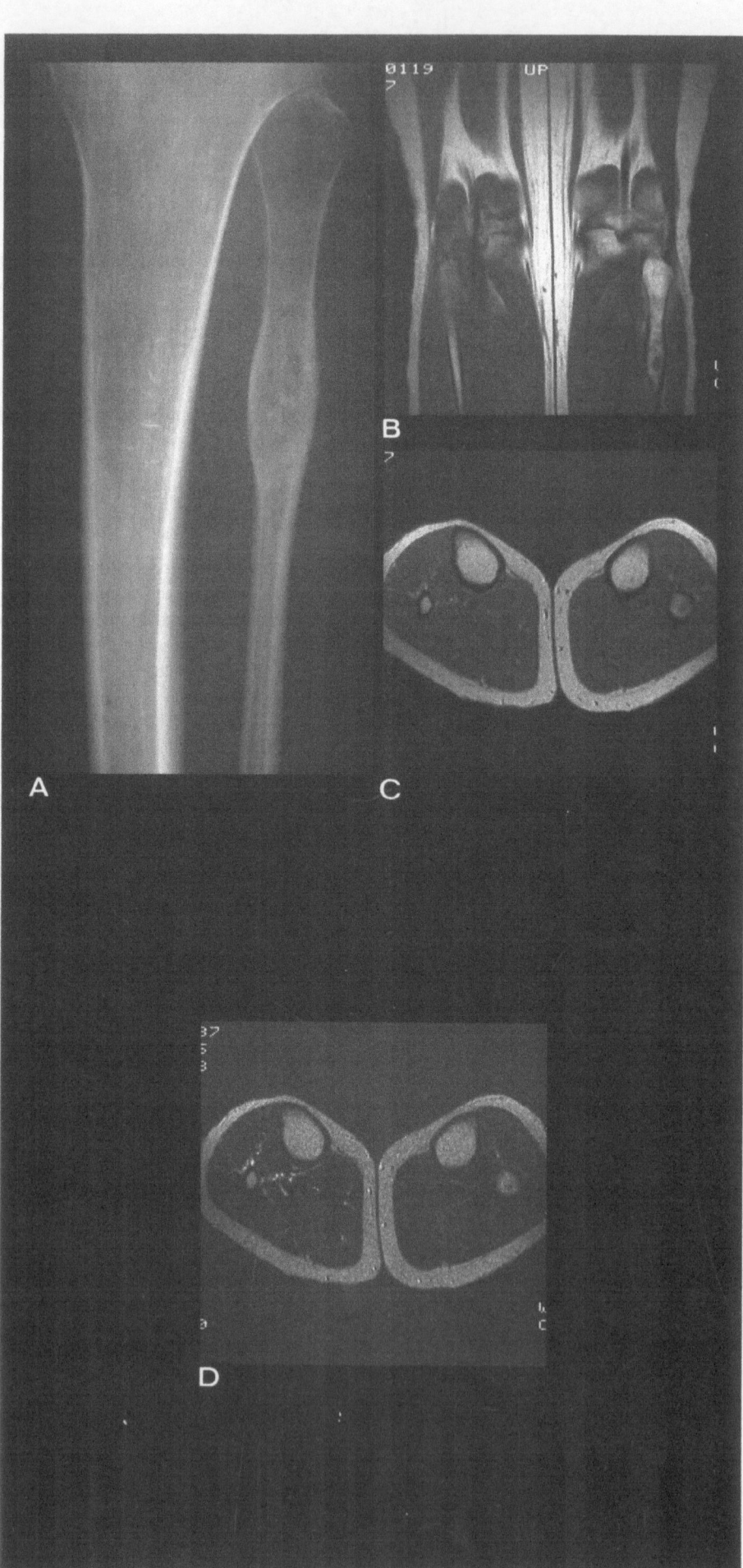

Fig. 4.1. B.M., 4l year-old female.

4.1.a. CR of the left lower leg.
Slightly radiolucent lesion at the
proximal third of the left fibula, causing
cortical expansion, endosteal scalloping
and containing central flecky
calcifications.

4.1.b. MRI of the lower legs, coronal
section, T1-WI.
Cocardelike lesion in the left fibula,
nearly isointense to normal marrow
[5] [6] with central signal void due to
intratumoral calcifications.

4.1.c and d. MRI of the lower legs,
transverse section, proton density-(c)
and T2-WI (d).
Here also the lesion has about the
same SI as adjacent normal marrow
[5] [6]. Central calcifications generate
no signal.

Diagnosis: Biopsy-proven enchondroma.

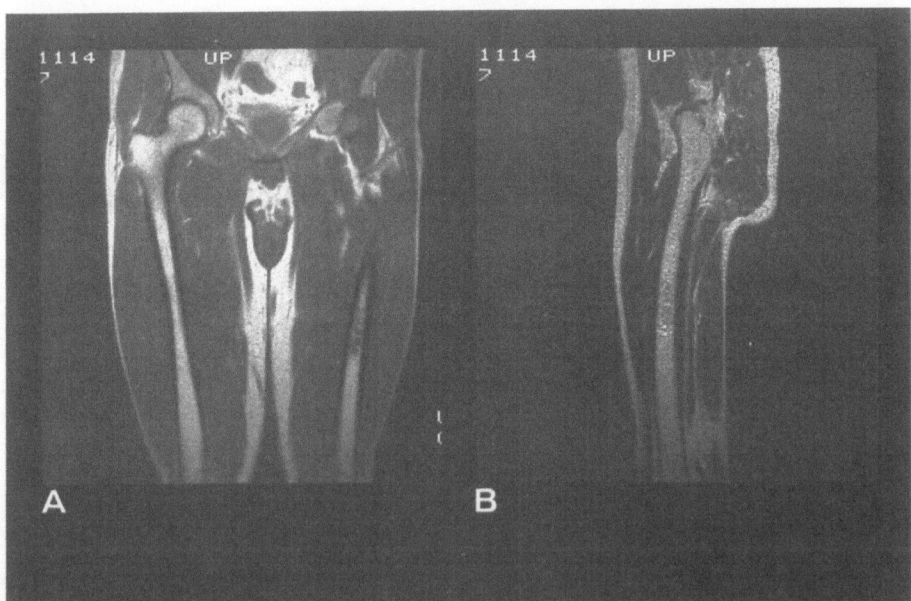

Fig. 4.2. D.V.M., 58 year-old male.

4.2.a. MRI of the left femur, coronal
section, T1-WI.
Mottled area of decreased SI in the
middle third of the diaphysis of the
left femur.

4.2.b. MRI of the left femur, sagittal
section, T2-WI.
Here also the lesion has a decreased SI.
Small foci of increased SI probably
represent cystic components.
Cortical bone remains intact on both
SE-sequences.

Diagnosis: Characteristic morphology and
SI of a mature medullary bone infarct.

Fig. 4.3. D.R., 57 year-old female.

4.3.a. CT at knee level, bone window.
Large, well circumscribed slightly
radiolucent lesion with serpiginous,
sclerotic margins at the distal
metaphysis of the right femur.

4.3.b. MRI of the knee region, coronal
section, T1-WI.
The lesion is demarcated by a low
SI serpiginous ring, due to reactive
interface.
Central area is inhomogeneous and
also of low SI.

4.3.c. MRI of the knee region, transverse
section, T2-WI.
Again the lesion presents with a
mainly low SI. Small foci of higher SI
probably represent areas of cystification.
The periphery of the lesion is of higher
SI, corresponding to reactive tissue.
Intraarticular high SI-line is due to an
associated minimal joint effusion
(curved arrows).

Diagnosis: Biopsy-proven mature bone
infarct.

34

CHAPTER 5

OSTEOCHONDROMA

Osteochondroma or osteocartilaginous exostosis is the most common
benign tumor of bone. It may be solitary or multiple (hereditary multiple
exostoses). The tumor manifests itself during adolescence or childhood.
There is no difference in sex incidence. Metaphysis of long tubular bones
is the most common localization.

Pathologically osteochondroma may be sessile or pedunculated. It is covered
with periosteum which is continuous with that of the adjacent cortical
bone. The surface of the exostosis is covered with a layer of hyaline
cartilage. The younger the patient, the more prominent the cartilage cap.
The growth of an osteochondroma usually ceases at puberty together with
fusion of the adjacent growth plate. At that moment the cap ossifies. On
occasion remnants of a quiescent cartilage cap may persist far into adult
life. The presence of a cap confirms the potential for further growth of
the tumor. If cap thickness exceeds 10 mm. one must be aware of
chondrosarcomatous change.

On MRI osteochondroma present with typical continuity of native cortex
and medullary cavity. The marrow of an osteochondroma is usually fatty
with corresponding SI (high SI in T1-WI, relatively high SI on T2-WI).
The cartilage cap may consist of lobules or lobules in lobules composed
of pure hyaline cartilage, generating a uniform, high SI on T2-WI and a
low SI on T1-WI. Lobules are defined by septa of low SI on both T1- and
T2-WI. A superficial zone of low SI may cover the cartilage cap,
corresponding to an intact perichondrium (1) (2) (3).

References

1. Cohen EK, Kressel HY, Frank TS, Fallon M et all. Hyaline cartilage-origin bone
   and soft-tissue neoplasms: MR appearance and histologic correlation. Radiology
   1988; 167: 477-481.
2. Lee JK, Yao L, Wirth CR. MR imaging of solitary osteochondromas: report of
   eight cases. AJR 1987; 149: 557-560.
3. Murphy WA, Totty WG. Musculoskeletal magnetic resonance imaging. Magnetic
   Resonance Annual 1986. edited by Herbert Y. Kressel. Raven Press,New York.

COMMENT

1. High SI exostotic cartilage cap (T2-WI) is seen in patients before the cessation of bone growth or when remnants of quiescent cartilage persist. Absence of the cap marks the end of exostotic growth. The high SI cap was seen in three of our five cases of osteochondroma. In one patient a thin cartilage cap was missed by MRI.

2. The presence of lobules, lobules in lobules, and septa within osteochondromas as reported in MR-literature, is noted in only one of our cases. Continuity of the medullary cavity, cortex, and/or perichondrium was demonstrated in all five cases. Dense exostotic mineralization, noted on plain radiographs, is seen on MRI as areas of signal absence, intervening between the higher signal area of the cartilage cap and the high signal medullary cavity (fatty marrow).

3. We used contrast medium in only one case. There was no enhancement on T1-WI after intravenous injection of Gadolinium DTPA. This is probably due to the poor vascularization of hyaline cartilage.
To the best of our knowledge no MR-contrast studies of osteochondromas are reported in the literature.

4. Extension of the osteochondroma is mostly equally well demonstrated by CT as by MRI (allowing for a radical surgical excision and hence preventing recurrence of the tumor). The role of MRI is mainly situated in detection and measurement of the hyaline cartilage cap.

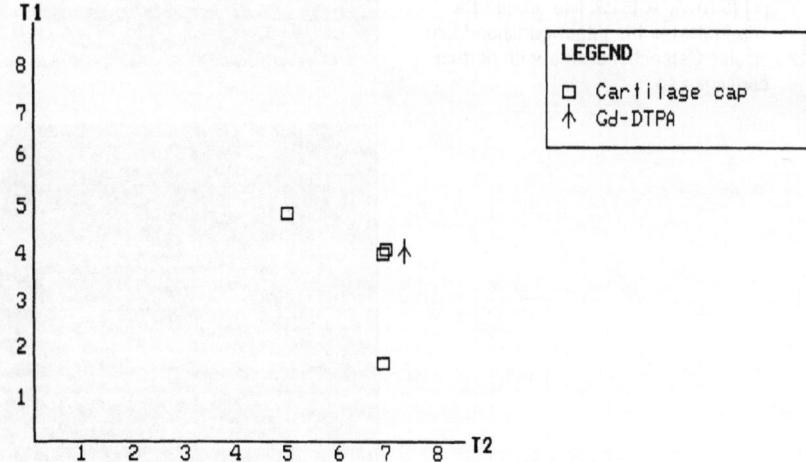

36

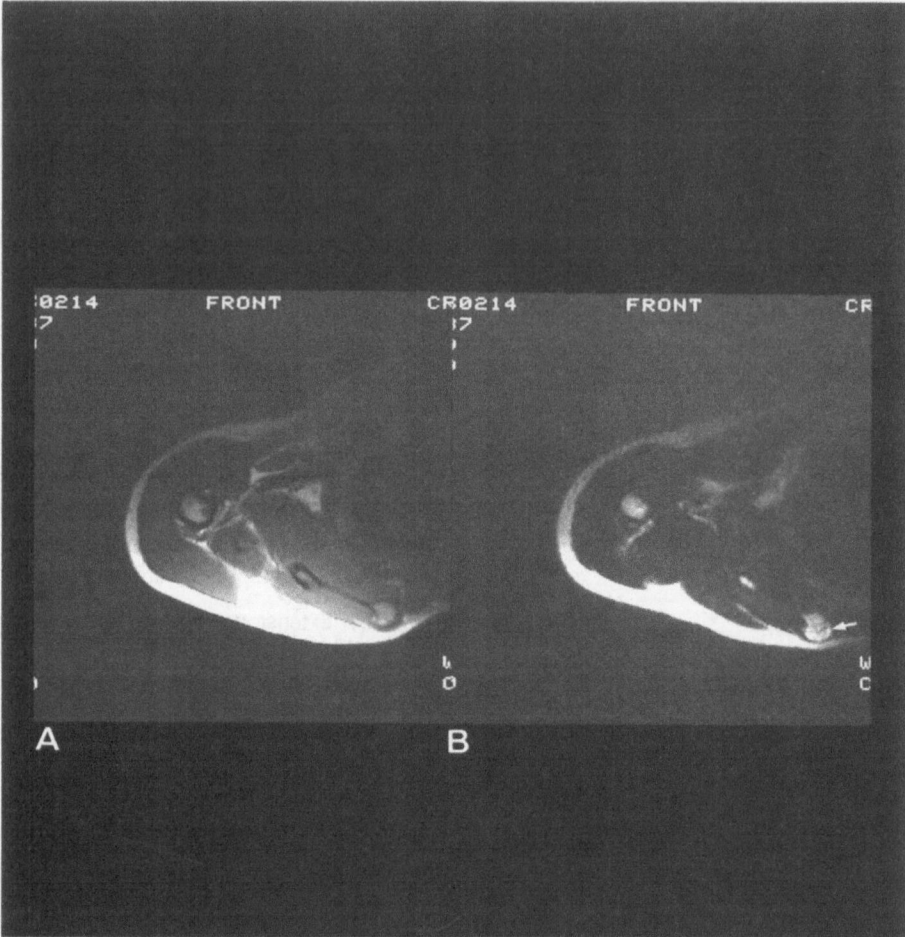

Fig. 5.1. V.G.E., 15 year-old female.

5.1.a. MRI of the right shoulder, transverse
section T1-WI.
Solitary osteochondroma at the medial
margin of the right scapula.
The central area of the lesion mass
has a relatively high SI [6] due to the
continuing medullary cavity (fatty
marrow). The peripheral cartilage cap
has a low SI [2].
5.1.b. MRI of the right shoulder, transverse
section T2-WI.
The central area of the lesion again
has the SI of fatty marrow. The clearly
delineated cartilage cap has a high SI
[7] (arrow). A black line around the
cap indicates the intact perichondrium.
Diagnosis: Osteochondroma with normal
cartilage cap.

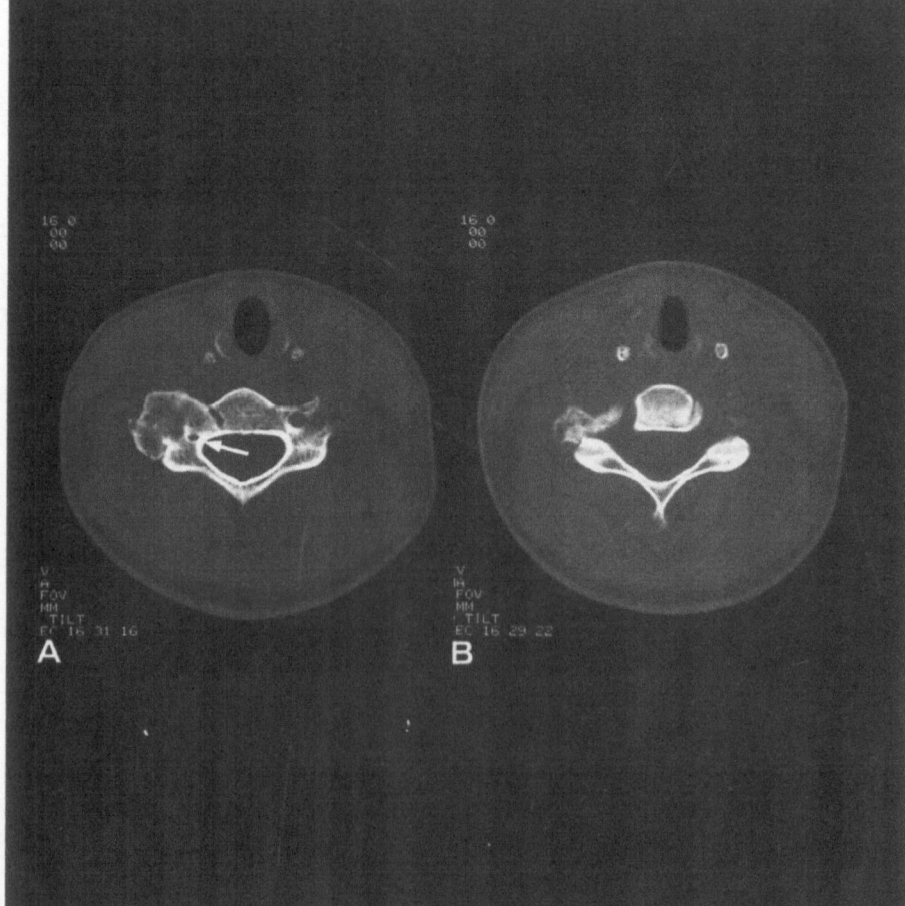

Fig. 5.2. A.C., 25 year-old female.

5.2.a. CT of the cervical spine, bone
window.
Exostosis of the right articular pillar
of C VI. Narrowing of the right
transverse foramen (arrow).
5.2.b. CT of the cervical spine, bone
window.
Section through the top of the
exostosis, extending towards the right
intervertebral foramen of C V-VI
Hypotrophy of the right uncus of C VI.

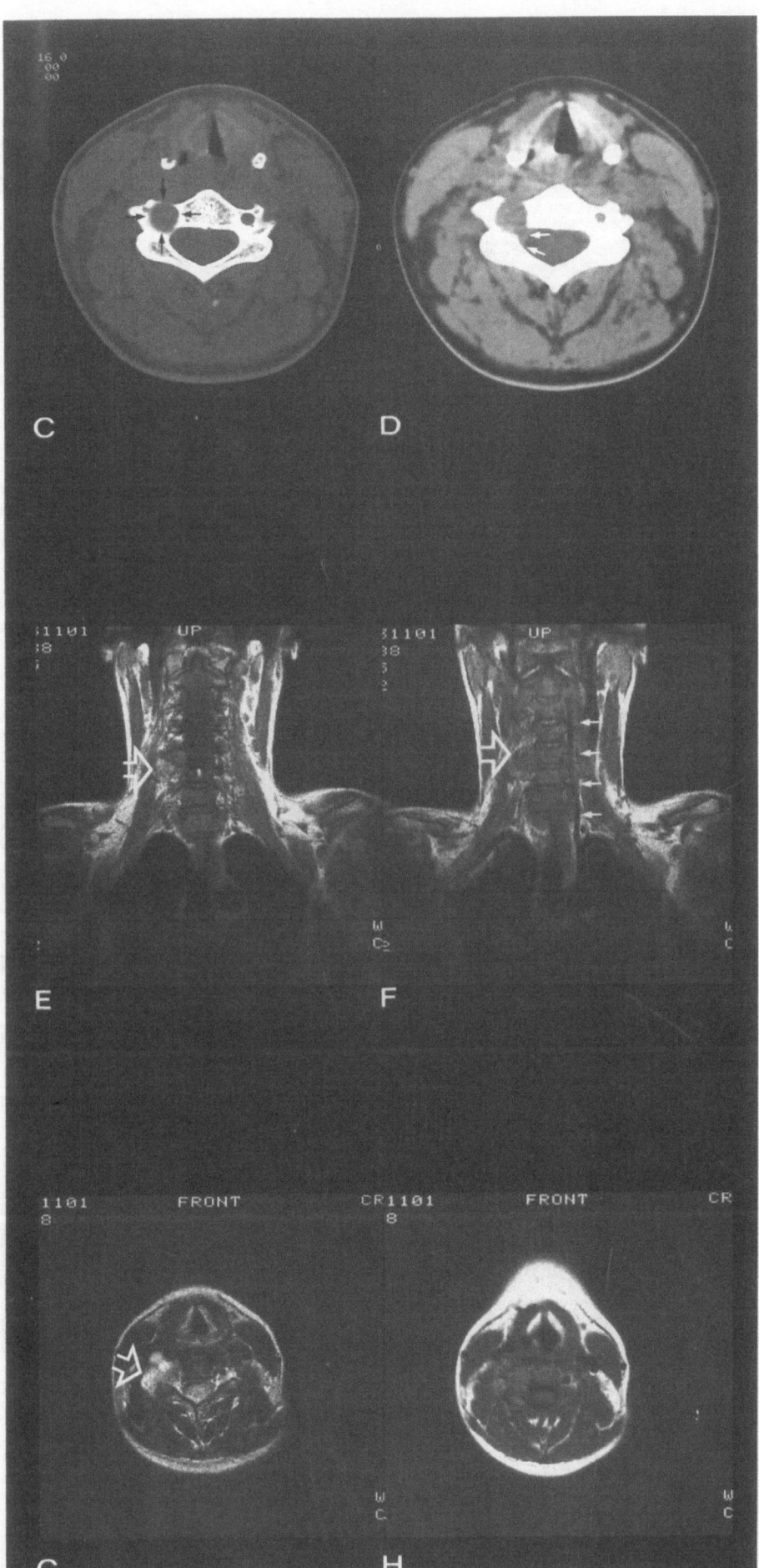

5.2.c. CT of the cervical spine, bone window.
Section through the body of C V with enlargement and ill delineation of the right transverse foramen of C V (arrows).

5.2.d. CT of the cervical spine, soft tissue window.
Soft tissue mass in the right transverse foramen of C V extending towards the vertebral canal (arrows).

5.2.e. MRI of the cervical spine, coronal section, T1-WI.
Lobulated mass on the right articular pillar of C V-VI (open arrow). The mass has a relatively high SI, probably due to the continuity of the medullary cavity (fatty marrow) into the exostosis.

5.2.f. MRI of the cervical spine, coronal section, T1-WI.
Section at the level of the transverse foramen of C V. The SI of the cranial part of the exostosis, extending into the transverse foramen of C V is definitely lower, probably due to the presence of a hyaline cartilage cap. Erosion of the lateral margin of C V (open arrow). Large left vertebral artery (small arrow) and no visible vertebral artery on the right side.

5.2.g. MRI of the cervical spine, transverse section, T2-WI.
Section at the same level as in Fig. 5.2.c. A lobulated mass with a high SI [7] represents the cartilage cap of the exostosis (open arrow).

5.2.h. MRI of the cervical spine, transverse section, T1-WI, after intravenous injection of Gd-DTPA.
There is no enhancement of the lesion.

Diagnosis: Osteochondroma with pathologically enlarged cartilage cap in a patient with known multiple exostoses.

38

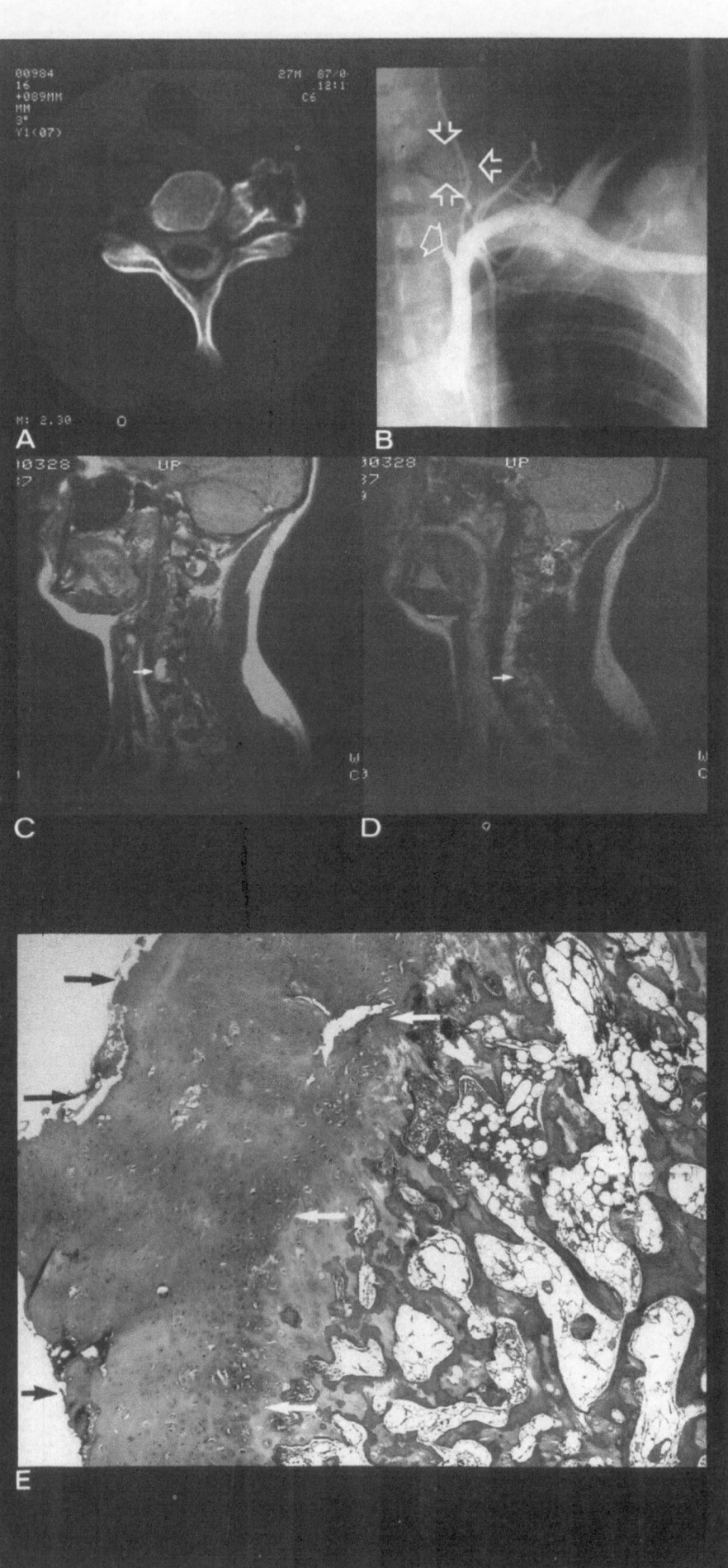

Fig. 5.3. R.E., 28 year-old male.

5.3.a. CT of the cervical spine after
intrathecal injection of contrast medium
(bone window).
Mushroomlike shaped osteochondroma
at the left articular pillar of C VII.
Low density of the central part of the
lesion and pronounced calcification
of the peripheral cap.

5.3.b. Angiography of the left subclavian
artery.
Cut-off at the proximal segment of
the left vertebral artery (large open
arrow), caused by extension of the
exostosis (open arrows) into the
transverse foramen.

5.3.c. MRI of the cervical spine, sagittal
section, T1-WI.
High SI of the central part and low
SI of the periphery of the lesion (arrow).

5.3.d. MRI of the cervical spine, sagittal
section, T2-WI.
Intermediate SI of the central part and
again low SI of the periphery.

5.3.e. Microphotograph of the resected
specimen.
The mass is limited by a small rim of
newly formed hyaline cartilage which
at the base shows endochondral
ossification (arrows).

Diagnosis: Osteochondroma with thin
cartilage cap, not detected by MRI.

CHAPTER 6

GIANT CELL TUMOR

Giant cell tumors represent 14-20% of all primary bone tumors. Both sexes are equally affected. They occur mostly after skeletal maturation. 50% of the tumors are located in the knee region. In cases of postoperative local recurrence, the tendency to malignancy is increased (10 to 20%).

Giant cell tumors consist of spindle-shaped and ovoid cells uniformly interspersed with multinucleated giant cells. Intratumoral necrosis and hemorrhage are often noted.

According to Sanerkin (2) the grading of giant cell tumors of bone is as follows:
1) Conventional tumors (86%) (grade I and II of Lichtenstein) with none of the features characterizing malignant or borderline tumors
2) Borderline tumors (9%) (grade II of Lichtenstein) without frank sarcomatous changes, but showing abnormal mitoses or vascular permeation or both
3) Malignant tumors (5%) (grade III of Lichtenstein) with frank sarcomatous changes and full metastatic potential.
The aggressiveness of giant cell tumors can not be ascertained on the basis of histologic criteria but is a clinical and radiological grading. Metastatic potential is low.

Radiologically giant cell tumors present as osteolytic lesions with poorly defined borders and an intermediate transition area. They are mostly eccentrically located in the epi-metaphysis of the long bones. Cortical permeation and cortical expansion are common signs. Periosteal new bone formation is almost absent. An accompanying soft tissue extension is often seen. Giant cell tumors frequently show signs of aggressiveness on CR-CT.

Only isolated cases of giant cell tumors examined by MRI are reported in the literature.
MR-findings reflect CR-CT features, SI-changes being aspecific in these cases (1).

References

1. Richardson ML, Kilcoyne RF, Gillespy III T, Helms CA, Genant HK. Magnetic resonance imaging of musculoskeletal neoplasms. Radiol Clin North Am 1986; 24(2): 259-267.
2. Sanerkin NG. Malignancy, aggressiveness and recurrence in giant cell tumor of bone. Cancer 1980; 46: 1641-1649.

COMMENT

1. Four patients with giant cell tumor were studied with MRI. All cases, with exception of the vertebral-extradural located tumor, presented with characteristic signs on CR-CT. All tumors had a CT-density comparable to normal muscle. Soft tissue extension was found only in one case.

2. MRI confirmed the characteristic morphological findings of CR-CT-studies, with exception of information about tumor extension in coronal-sagittal plane. (i.e. extension to diaphyseal area and adjacent joints).

3. All lesions had an intermediate SI on both T1- and T2-WI, except for the soft tissue component of the vertebral giant cell tumor, which had a high SI [8] on T2-WI.

4. In two cases Gd-DTPA was injected. A uniform but moderate enhancement was noted in both cases.

5. It was not possible on the basis of morphological or SI-information to differentiate between the different histological types of giant cell tumor. On the contrary, aggressiveness and extent of these tumors were more easily ascertained by MRI than by histology.

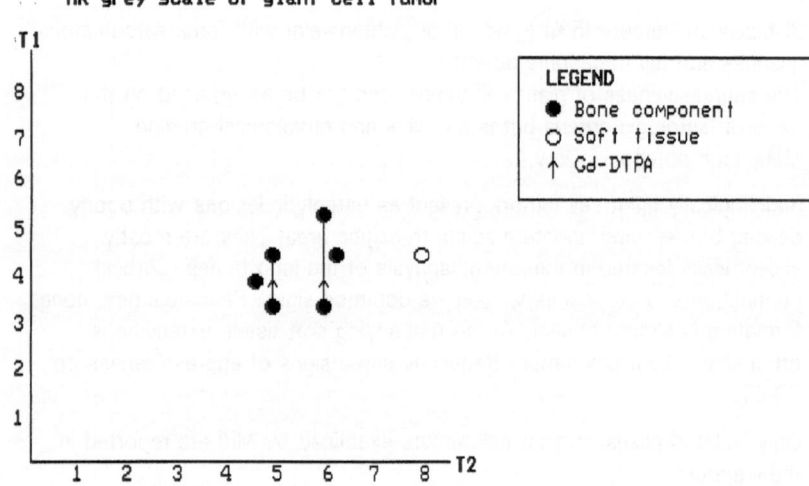

MR-grey scale of giant cell tumor

LEGEND
● Bone component
○ Soft tissue
↑ Gd-DTPA

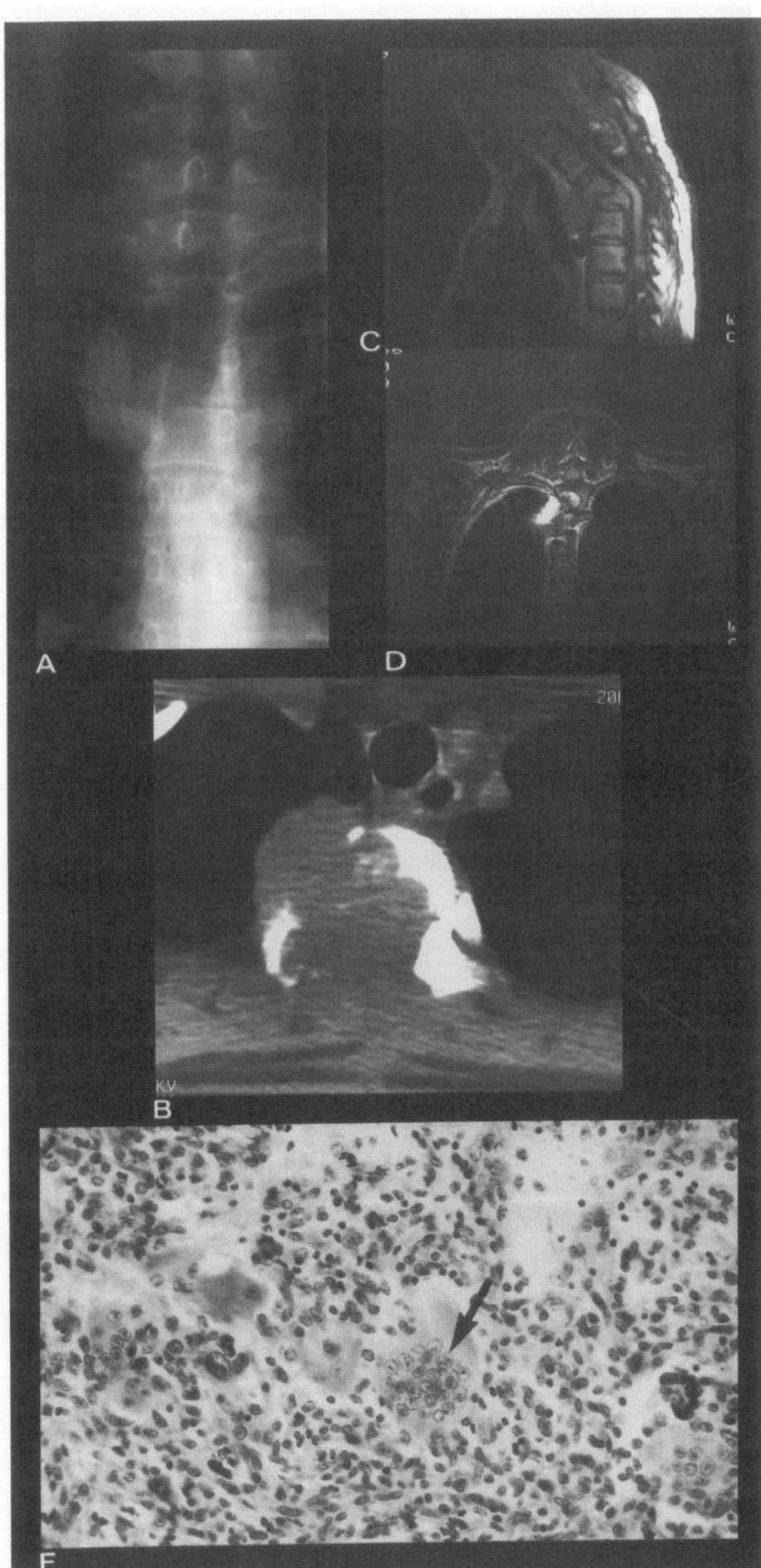

Fig. 6.1. W.M., 24 year-old female.

6.1.a. CR of the thoracic spine.
Destructive lesion of vertebra TH III
with accompanying soft tissue mass
responsible for broadening of the
mediastinum.

6.1.b. CT (soft tissue window) of the
thoracic spine at the level of TH III.
Confirmation of the destructive lesion
at TH III with extension to the posterior
mediastinum and the spinal canal.
The tumor has a mean density
comparable to normal muscle.

6.1.c. MRI of the cervical spine, sagittal
section, T1-WI.
The sagittal image clearly demonstrates
the ventrally located soft tissue mass,
the extensive destruction-compression
of TH III and the posterior extension
with displacement and compression
of the spinal cord. Both bone and
soft tissue components have an
intermediate SI [4] [5].

6.1.d. MRI of the cervical spine, coronal
section, T2-WI.
The full extent of the lesion is difficult
to evaluate due to the extensive
kyphosis of the thoracic spine. Bony
as well as soft tissue components
are relatively sharply demarcated and
show an intermediate [6] (bone)
(arrows) to high [8] (soft tissue) SI.

6.1.e. Microphotograph (Courtesy Prof
J.J.Martin, UZA).
Numerous multinucleated giant cells,
amidst many mononucleated cells
(arrow).

Diagnosis: Giant cell tumor, type I.

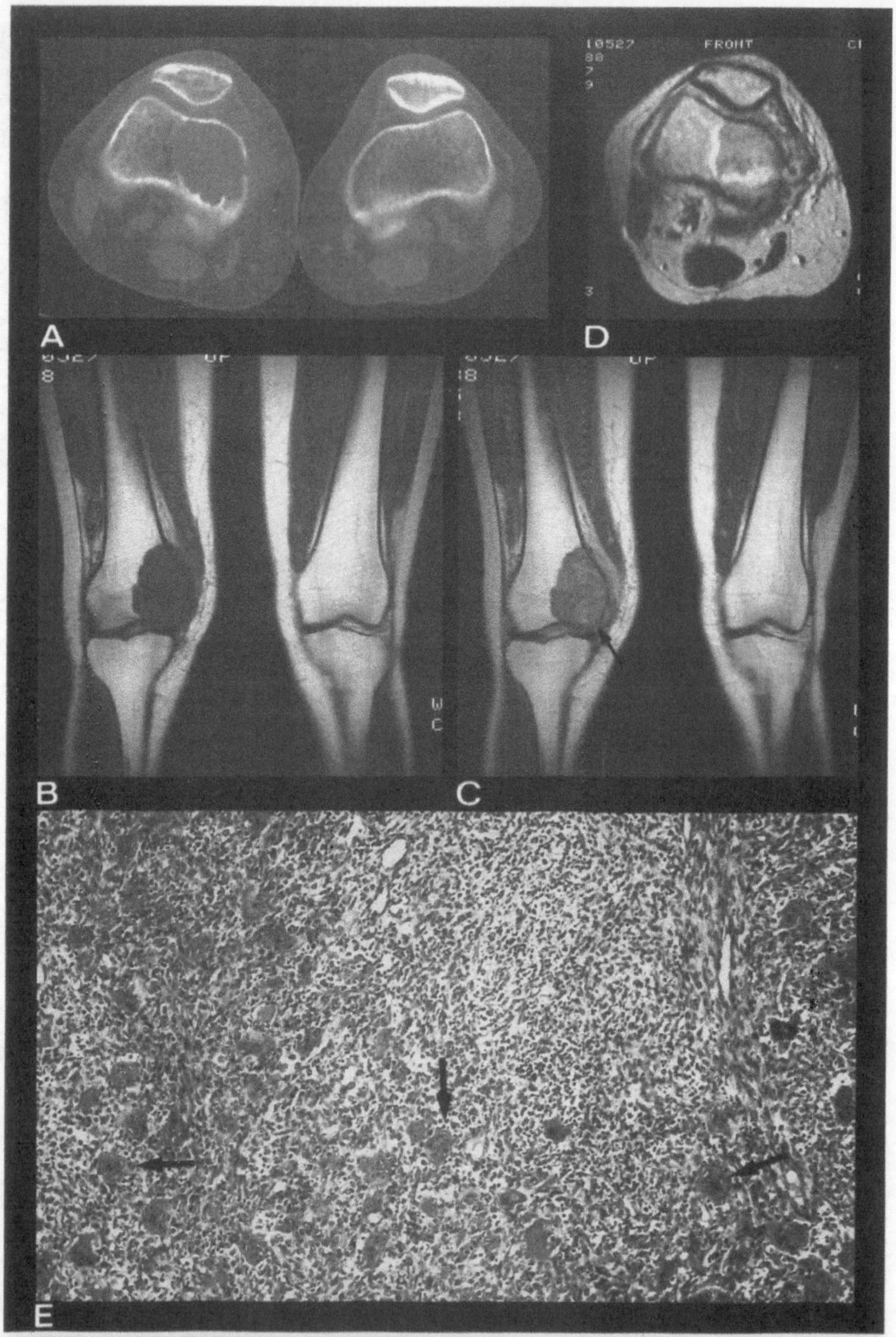

42

Fig. 6.2. P.I., 45 year-old female.

6.2.a. CT at knee level.
Eccentric, osteolytic lesion at the distal epi-metaphysis of the right femur. Moderate cortical expansion and disruption at the medial margin. Homogeneous aspect of the lesion and mean density comparable to normal muscle.

6.2.b and c. MRI at knee level, coronal section, T1-WI before (b) and after (c) intravenous injection of Gd-DTPA.
b. Sharp demarcation of the lesion with SI comparable to SI of normal muscle [3] [4] and low SI peripheral rim. Adjacent hyaline cartilage at the medial femoral condyle remains intact.
c. Moderate enhancement after contrast injection. Cocardelike central image is due to previous biopsy (arrow).

6.2.d. MRI of the knee, transverse section, T2-WI.
Less homogeneous aspect of the lesion with an intermediate SI [5]. High SI of the peripheral rim.

6.2.e. Microphotograph.
Numerous giant cells in a stroma of spindle-shaped cells (arrows).

Diagnosis: Characteristics of a conventional giant cell tumor, type I.

Fig. 6.3. S.W., 36 year-old female.

6.3.a. MRI of the left forearm, coronal section, T1-WI.
Large, bilobated lesion at the distal epi-metaphysis of the left radius extending to the radiocarpal joint. Cortical expansion and destruction. Narrow zone of transition with adjacent diaphyseal marrow. The lesion has an intermediate and quite uniform SI [3] [4]. Note also the difference in SI between the proximal and distal part of the left scaphoid (arrow).

6.3.b. MRI of the left forearm, coronal section, T1-WI, after intravenous injection of Gd-DTPA.
There is marked homogeneous enhancement of the lesion. At the level of the scaphoid bone there is no enhancement of the distal part compared to the proximal part (arrow).

Diagnosis: Histologically borderline type of giant cell tumor.
Ischemic necrosis of the scaphoid bone.

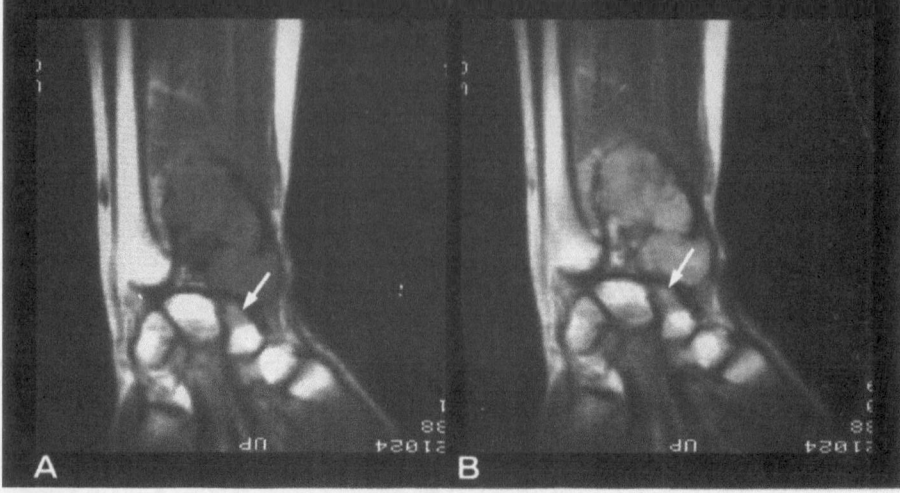

43

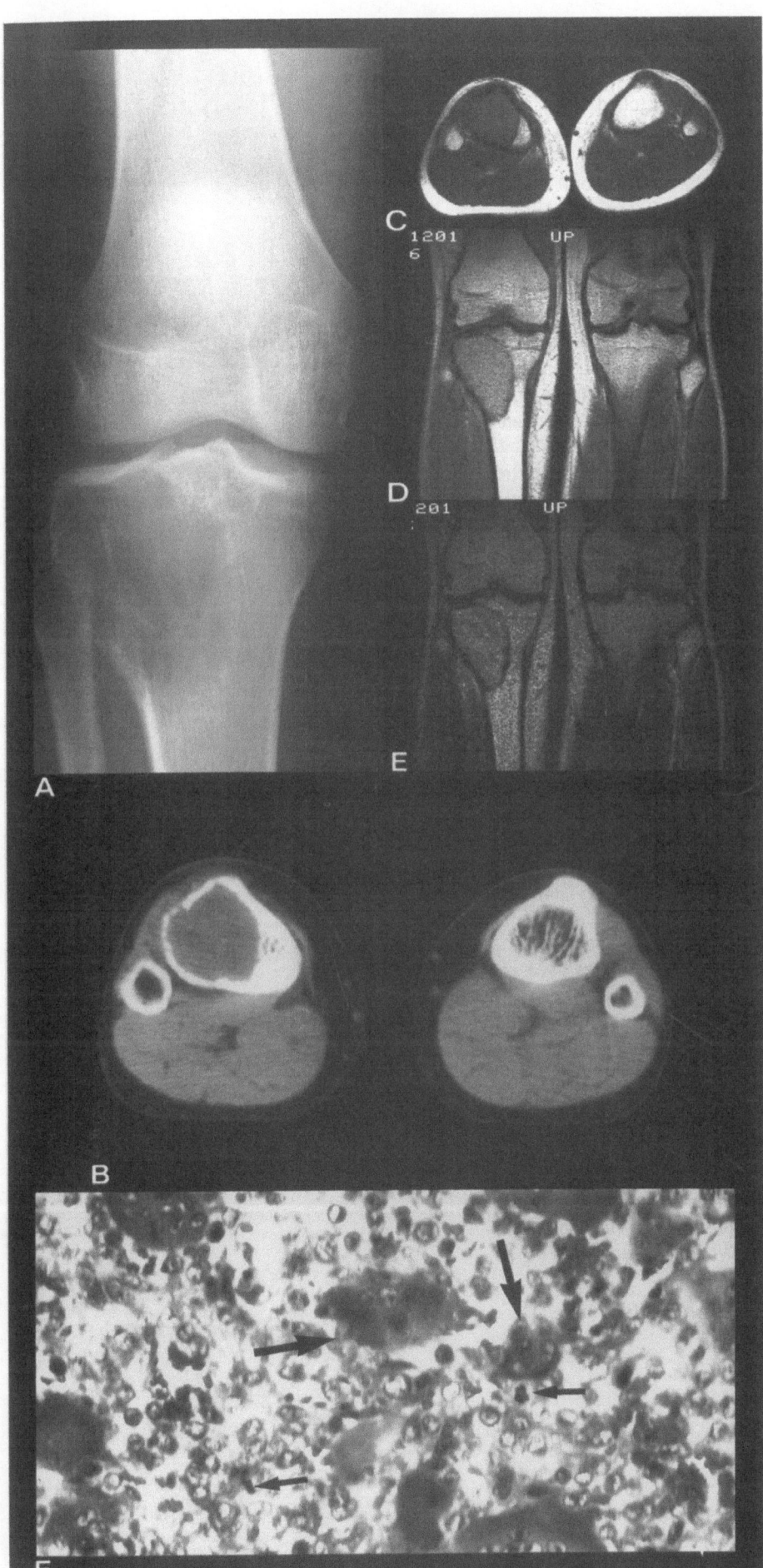

Fig. 6.4. D.P., 20 year-old male.

6.4.a. CR of the right knee.
Eccentrically located osteolytic lesion at the proximal epi-metaphysis of the right tibia. Cortical expansion and disruption at the lateral margin.

6.4.b. CT at knee level.
Confirmation of CR-findings. No visible soft tissue component. Homogeneous aspect of the lesion. The mean density is comparable to the density of normal muscle.

6.4.c. MRI of the knee, transverse section, T1-WI.
Homogeneous aspect of the lesion which is sharply demarcated by a small line of low SI. (narrow zone of transition)."Dirty" appearance of the lateral cortical bone. Cortical disruption is less evident on MRI compared to combined CR-CT.

6.4.d and e. MRI of the knee, coronal section, proton density-(d) and T2-WI (e).
Again the mass is homogeneous and sharply demarcated by a low SI-rim. The exact localization, the full extent and the relationship to the adjacent normal knee joint are clearly demonstrated on these coronal sections. Uniform and intermediate to high SI [5] of the lesion.

6.4.f. Microphotograph (Courtesy Dr.Van Strijthem, Antwerp).
Numerous giant cells (long arrows). Abnormal mitotic figures (short arrows).

Diagnosis: Giant cell tumor, borderline type.

44

CHAPTER 7

HEMANGIOMA

Hemangiomas are benign hamartomas most commonly found in the
calvarium and the vertebral bodies. The highest incidence is found in middle
aged and elderly women.
Hemangiomas may be capillary or cavernous. In the capillary form there
is a radiating intraosseus capillary network. In the cavernous form large
sinuses and vessels cause resorption of bone trabeculae.
There are two types of vertebral hemangioma. The first one is
asymptomatic and incidentally found on conventional radiographs or CT.
The second rare one is responsible for slowly progressive compression
of the spinal cord (3).
Characteristic features by which compressive vertebral hemangiomas can
be distinguished from asymptomatic vertebral hemangioma were described
by Laredo (1). Compressive vertebral hemangiomas are located between
TH III and TH IX, they present with involvement of the entire vertebral
body, extension to the neural arch (particularly pedicles), expanded cortex
with indistinct margins, irregular honeycomb pattern and soft-tissue mass.
Asymptomatic vertebral hemangiomas are mostly situated in the lumbar
spine, with complete or partial involvement of the vertebral body, a regular
striated or honeycomb appearance and well defined margins. Angiography
showed an almost normal vascularization in the asymptomatic group and
a hypervascularization in the compressive group.

A differential diagnosis has to be made between the compressive type of
vertebral hemangioma and Paget's disease or metastasis.

Ross J. (4) reports the MR-findings of ten vertebral hemangiomas in 8
patients. He describes a mottled increased SI of the osseous portion of
the tumor on T1- and T2-WI while the extraosseous components of the
tumor failed to demonstrate an increased SI on T1-WI but have an increased
SI on T2-WI. Increased SI on T1-WI is due to adipose tissue in the osseous
tumor which is absent in the extraosseous component. Fat attenuation
was confirmed by CT, and fat was demonstrated histologically. Only one
vertebral hemangioma in Ross series belongs to the compressive type. In
this case MR showed a very fine mottling of signal on T1- and T2-WI.
Blood flow contributes little to the T1-SI at the pulse sequences used
because of different SI of the osseous and the extra-osseous tumor
component which have the same vascularization pattern.
The exact cause of the increased SI on T2-WI may be tumor hypercellularity
but remains a matter of speculation.
In a personal communication Laredo distincts an inverted relation between
the amount of fat tissue and the amount of angiomatous tissue in vertebral
hemangiomas (2).
If a vertebral hemangioma has a high SI on T1-WI one can predict the
presence of a poorly vascularized lesion on angiography and the
hemangioma is mostly asymptomatic. The opposite is true for the
compressive type which lacks high SI on T1-WI and presents as an
hypervascular lesion on angiography.
To the best of our knowledge there are no reports of vertebral
hemangiomas studied by MR after contrast injection.

References

1. Laredo JD, Reizine D, Bard M, Merland JJ. Vertebral hemangiomas: radiologic
   evaluation. Radiology 1986; 161: 183-189.
2. Laredo JD Présentation Clinique et Classification des Hémangiomes Vertebraux.
   Personal communication 1988.
3. Leehey P, Naseem M, Every P, Russell E, Sarwar M. Vertebral hemangioma with
   compression myelopathy: metrizamide CT demonstration. J Comput Assist
   Tomogr 1985; 9(5): 985-986.
4. Ross JS, Masaryk TJ, Modic MT, Carter JR, Mapstone T, Dengel FH. Vertebral
   hemangiomas: MR imaging. Radiology 1987; 165: 165-169.

COMMENT

1. Six patients with vertebral hemangioma were studied with MRI. Three patients were asymptomatic (incidental finding). Three patients presented with neurological symptoms. In these cases vertebral hemangiomas were detected by CR or CT.

2. Asymptomatic vertebral hemangiomas show no or minimal tracer fixation on RNSC. A definite hyperfixation was found in our three symptomatic patients.

3. In all three cases of asymptomatic vertebral hemangioma the height of the vertebral body was normal and no symptoms of epidural space or dural sac compressions were present.

4. In the symptomatic vertebral hemangiomas there was a consistent finding of vertebral body compression, intravertebral disc herniation, bulging of the posterior vertebral wall and/or involvement of the spinal canal or neural foramina.

5. Asymptomatic lesions constantly have a very high SI on T1-WI and an intermediate SI on T2-WI.

6. Conversely symptomatic lesions in our series had a low to intermediate SI on T1-WI and on intermediate SI on T2-WI.

7. Two cases of symptomatic hemangioma were studied after injection of Gd-DTPA. A slight enhancement was seen in both cases. This confirms the above mentioned statement of Laredo (2).

8. Differential diagnosis: another patient with a roughly striated vertebral bone appearance was referred for MRI with the presumed diagnosis of vertebral hemangioma. However, in this case SI was completely different compared to the findings in our series of vertebral hemangiomas. Subsequently the lesion was found to be an osteoblastic metastasis of a breast carcinoma (Fig 7.6).

9. MRI seems to be able to differentiate between the two types of vertebral hemangioma not only by the morphological appearance of the lesion but also by their characteristic SI. In this regard, MRI has a diagnostic, differential diagnostic and prognostic value. Since symptomatic vertebral hemangiomas need an appropriate treatment, MRI also has a therapy-planning value.

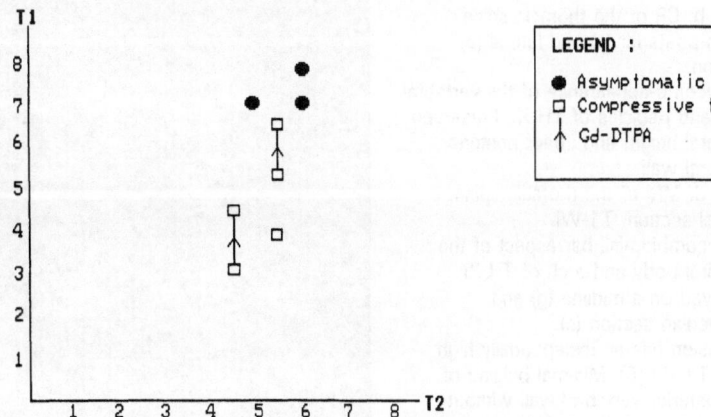

46

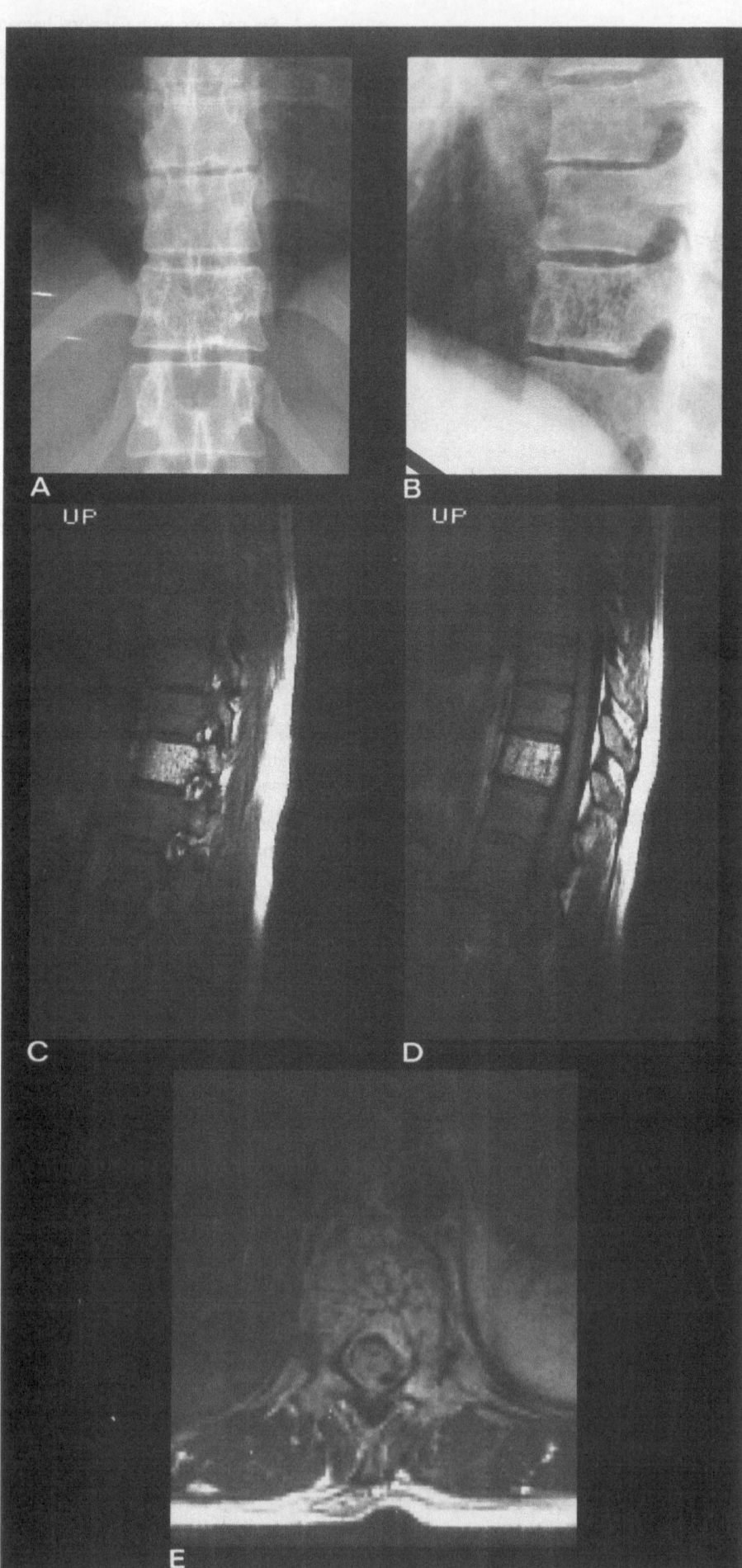

Fig. 7.1. V.D. 42 year-old female.

7.1.a and b. CR of the thoracic spine,
antero-posterior (a) and lateral (b)
position.
Honeycomb-appearance of the vertebral
body and pedicles of TH XI. Preserved
vertebral height and intact posterior
vertebral wall.

7.1.c and d. MRI of the thoracic spine,
sagittal section, T1-WI.
Honeycombing-jail bar aspect of the
vertebral body and arch of TH XI,
displayed on a midline (d) and
paramedian section (c).
The lesion has an exceptionally high
SI on T1-WI [8]. Minimal bulging of
the posterior vertebral wall without
compression of the dural sac and
spinal cord.

7.1.e. MRI of the thoracic spine, transverse
section, T2-WI.
The vertebral hemangioma has an
intermediate SI [5] on T2-WI.

Diagnosis: Example of an asymptomatic
vertebral hemangioma with characteristic
morphological appearance and SI on
MRI.

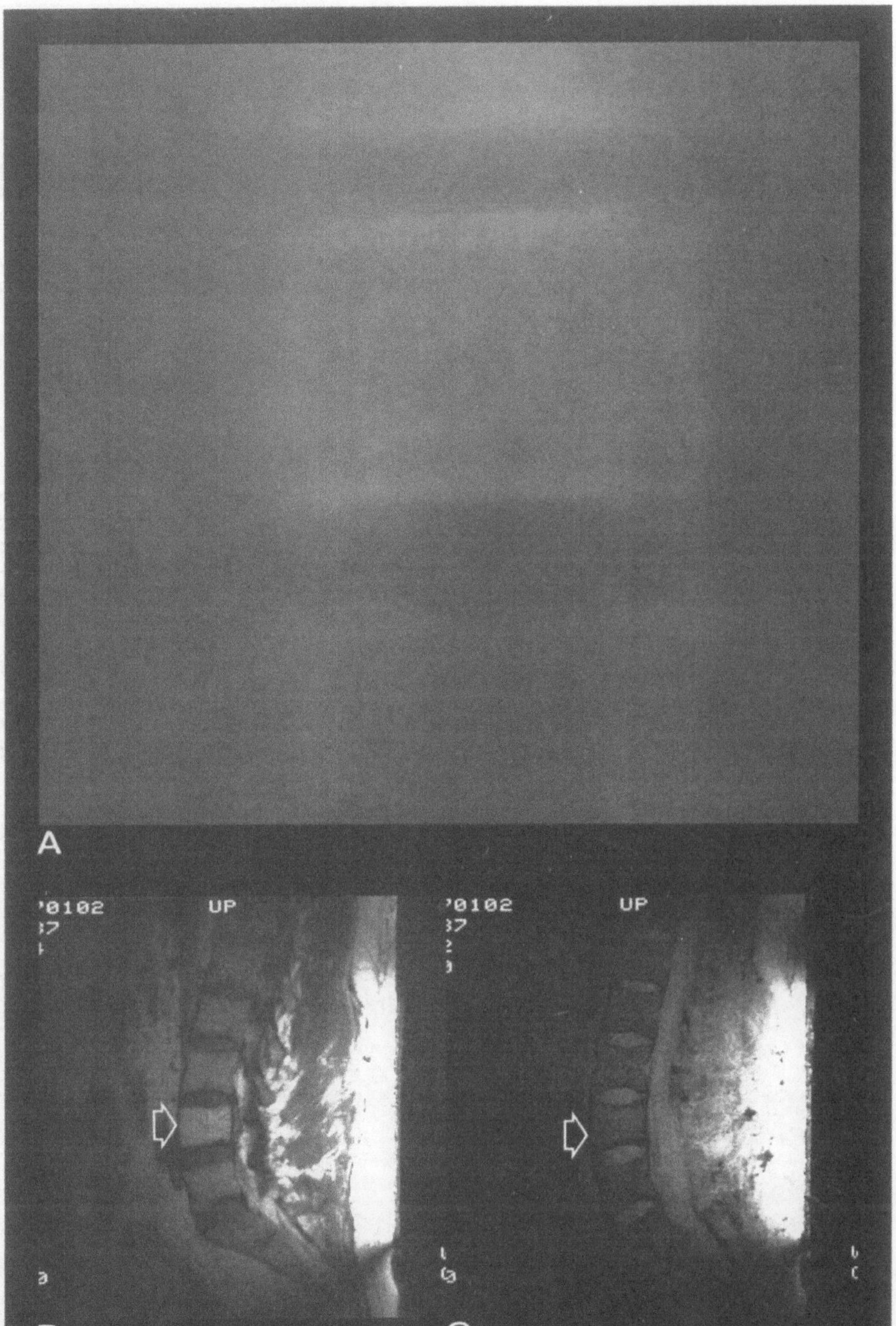

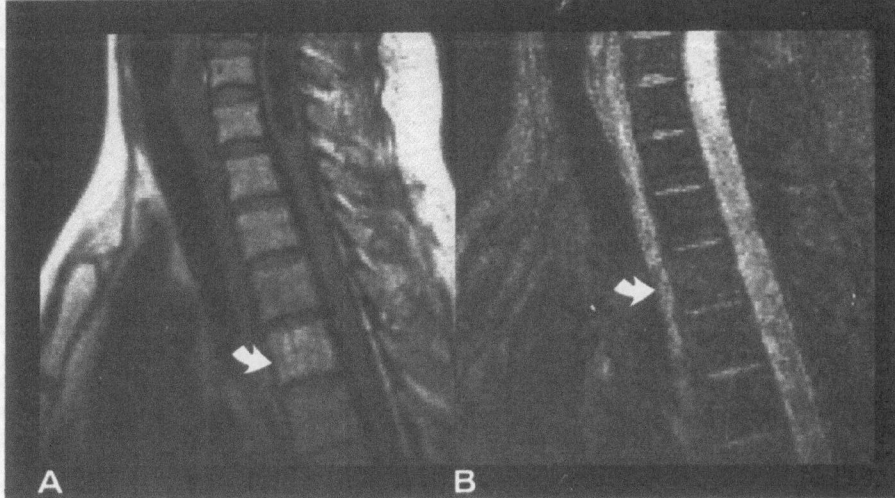

A

'0102   UP   '0102   UP

B   C

A   B

Fig. 7.2. D.M.T., 31 year-old male.

7.2.a. CR (tomography) of L IV.
   Striated appearance of the vertebral
   body of L IV. Vertebral height remains
   normal.
7.2.b. MRI at the level of L IV, transverse
   section, T1-WI.
   Uniform, high SI of the vertebral body
   (arrow). Slightly flattened posterior
   vertebral wall without impression on
   the epidural space or dural sac.
7.2.c. MRI at the level of L IV, transverse
   section, T2-WI.
   Striated aspect and intermediate SI
   of the vertebral body of L IV (arrow).
Diagnosis: Non compressive type of
   vertebral hemangioma.

Fig. 7.3. V.M.J., 59 year-old female.

7.3.a and b. MRI of the thoracic spine,
   sagittal section.
   Vertebral hemangioma of the vertebral
   body TH V with characteristic SI on
   a T1-WI (a) and a T2-WI (b) (arrow).
Diagnosis: Incidental discovery of an
   asymptomatic vertebral hemangioma
   in a patient with syringomyelia.

48

Fig. 7.4. S.A., 37 year-old male.

7.4.a and b. CR of the lumbar spine,
   antero-posterior (a) and lateral (b) view.
   a. Striated aspect of the vertebral
   body of L III.
   b. Displacement of the posterior
   vertebral wall with signs of bone
   resorption in the posterior part of the
   vertebral body and in the posterior
   elements of L III (pedicles, apophyseal
   joints and spinous process). Both
   diameters of the vertebral body are
   increased.
7.4.c. CT of the lumbar spine (L III), soft
   tissue window.
   Striated, honeycomb aspect of the
   whole vertebra L III. Narrowing of the
   spinal canal.
7.4.d. MRI of the lumbar spine, sagittal
   section, T1-WI.
   Bulging of the posterior wall of L III,
   compression of the epidural space
   and dural sac. Decreased SI [3] best
   demonstrated at the dorsal part of
   the vertebral body.
7.4.e. MRI, sagittal section, T1-WI after
   intravenous injection of Gd-DTPA.
   Moderate enhancement of the
   pathological vertebral body, arch and
   spinous process. SI is slightly higher
   than SI of adjacent vertebral bodies.
   Presence of intravertebral disc
   herniations.
7.4.f. MRI, sagittal section, T2-WI.
   Butterfly aspect of the vertebral body
   of L III due to intravertebral disc
   herniations. Intermediate SI [4] [5] of
   the vertebral body. Increased SI of
   the spinous process.
Diagnosis: Example of a symptomatic
   vertebral hemangioma. Bone resorption
   leads to vertebral compression (with
   intravertebral disc herniation) and
   concomitant protrusion of the posterior
   wall and narrowing of the spinal canal.

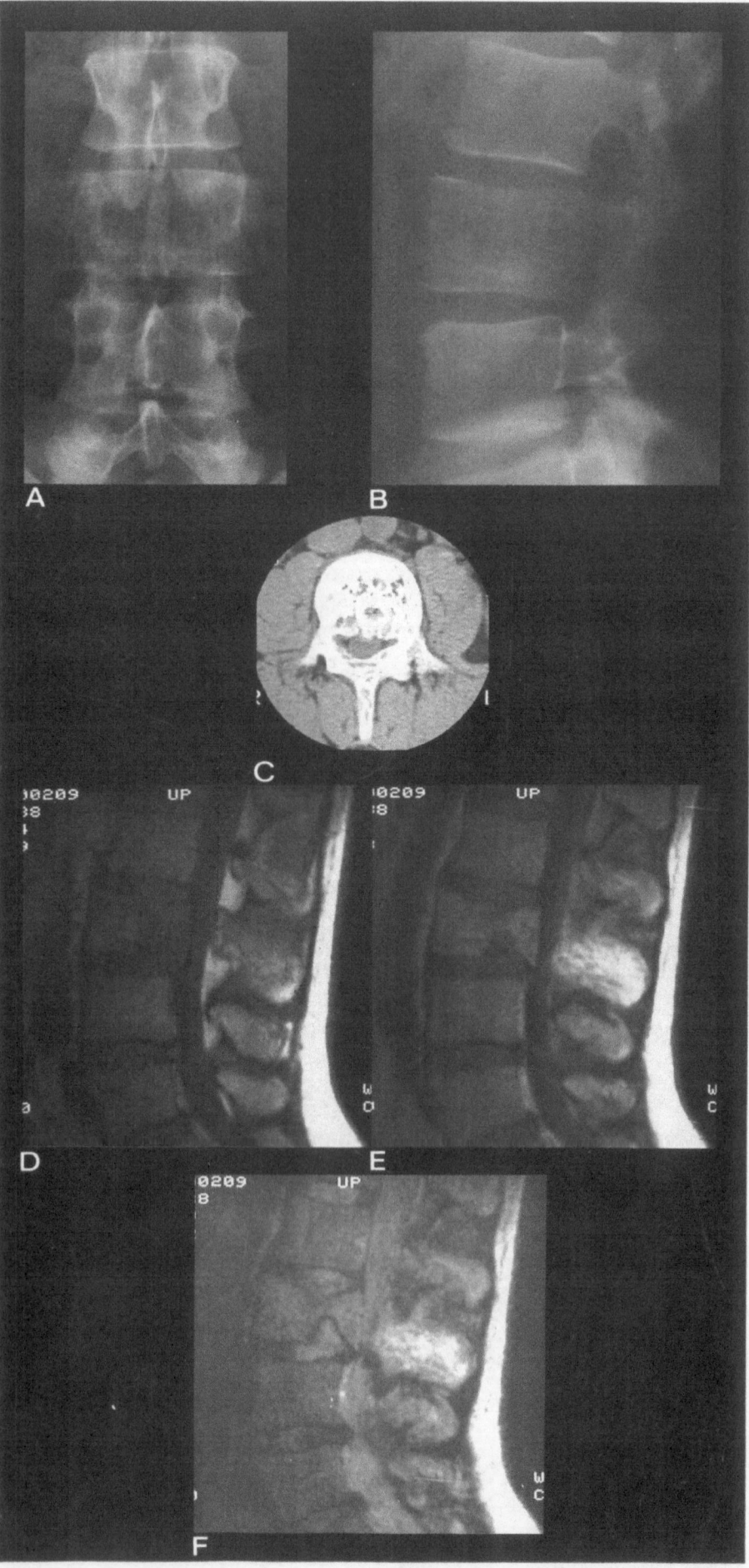

49

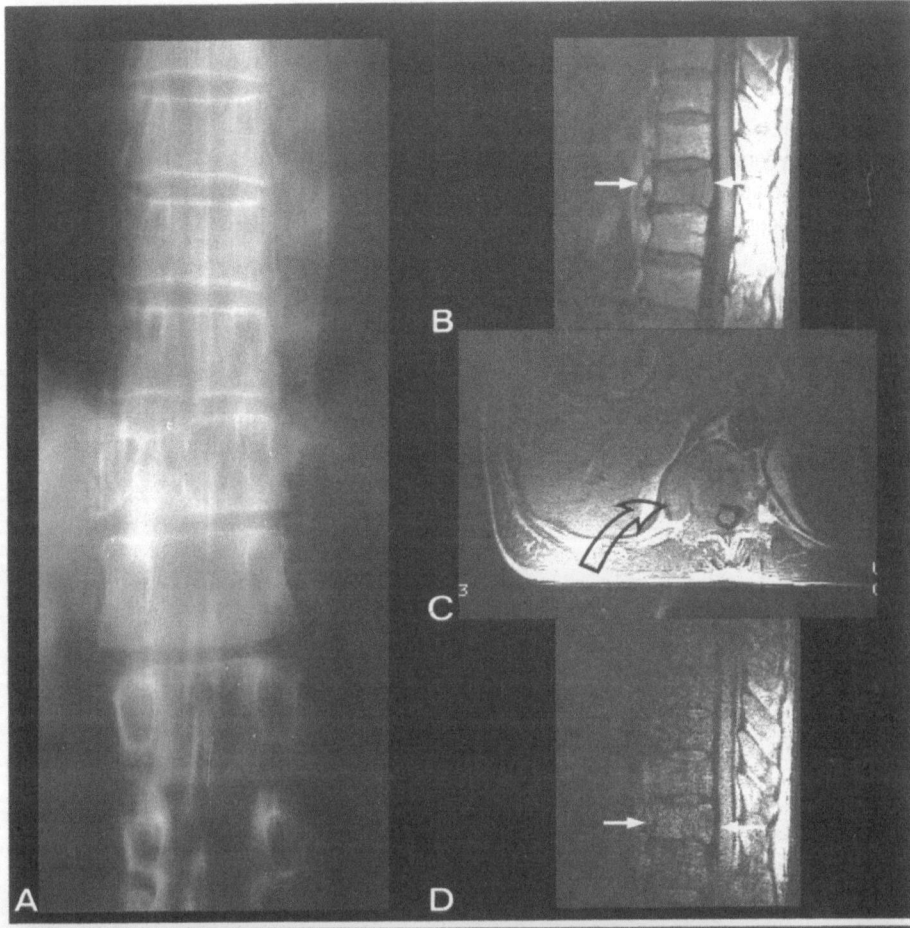

Fig. 7.5. V.L., 52 year-old male.

7.5.a. CR of the thoracic spine.
Striated aspect of vertebral body TH XII. Vertebral compression with increased latero-lateral diameter, and intravertebral disc herniations.
7.5.b. MRI, sagittal section, T1-WI.
Increased antero-posterior diameter of the vertebral body TH XII with bulging of the posterior wall and impression on the epidural space (arrows). The striated aspect is less obvious. Decreased SI [4] in comparison to adjacent vertebral bodies.
7.5.c. MRI, transverse section, T1-WI.
Paravertebral soft tissue component (curved open arrow) which is isointense to the pathological vertebral body.
7.5.d. MRI, sagittal section, T2-WI.
Pathological vertebral body has a slightly higher SI [5] [6] (arrow), compared to adjacent vertebrae.
Diagnosis: Compressive type of vertebral hemangioma.

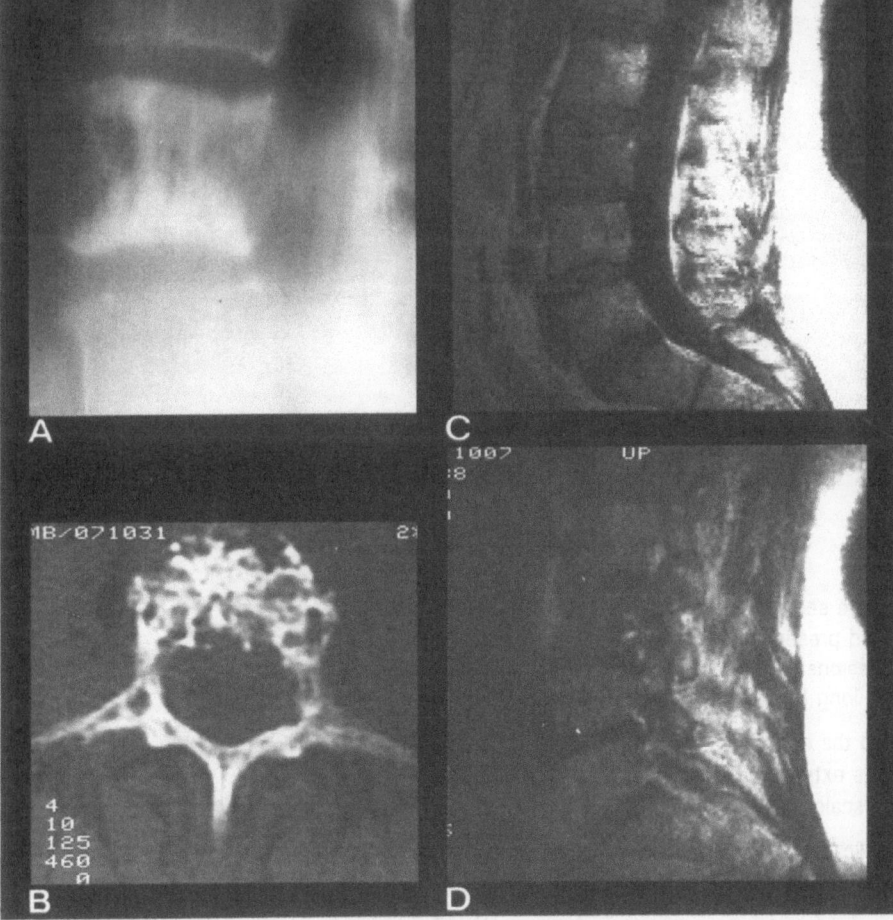

Fig. 7.6. N.T., 57 year-old female.

7.6.a. CR (tomography) of the lumbar spine. Roughly striated aspect of vertebral body L III.
7.6.b. CT of the lumbar spine.
Honeycomb or permeated appearance of L III. The lesion not only concerns the vertebral body but also vertebral pedicles, arch and processes.
7.6.c. MRI, sagittal section, T1-WI.
Patchy, inhomogeneous aspect and SI of all lumbar vertebrae.
7.6.d. MRI, sagittal section, T2-WI.
More uniform low SI of vertebral body L III.
Diagnosis: Osteoblastic metastasis of a breast carcinoma.

CHAPTER 8

SOLITARY BONE CYST

Solitary bone cysts are juvenile lesions (mean age 10 years) preferentially located in the proximal third of the humeral of femoral diaphysis. They rarely cause symptoms unless pathological fractures occur (Fig. 1.2).

Solitary bone cysts are fluid filled cavities delineated by a layer of cells resembling the cells of normal synovium, interspersed with fibrous and vascular tissue. Osteoid and osseous tissue as well as osteoclasts and multinucleated giant cells may be present.

Radiologically they present as radiolucent, sharply demarcated and trabeculated lesions, centrally located in the dia-metaphyseal region. Cortical broadening is more pronounced on the metaphyseal end of the lesion. On MRI simple cysts are lobulated, sharply demarcated lesions with a mean SI of muscle [3] on T1-WI and an extremely high SI [8] on T2-WI.

References: see chapter 9

COMMENT

1. Four cases of juvenile solitary bone cyst were seen in our series. Cysts were non complicated in three cases and present with the same morphological characteristics: multilobulated lesions separated by septa and located at the meta-diaphyseal regions of long bones.

2. SI on T1-WI was slightly different owing to the content of the lesion (less or more proteinaceous). SI on T2-WI was extremely high. Septa had a low SI on both SE-sequences. (for MR-grey scale, see chapter 9)

3. In one case a solitary bone cyst was complicated by a pathological fracture. Intracystic and periosteal hemorrhage were responsible for atypical morphological and SI-signs.

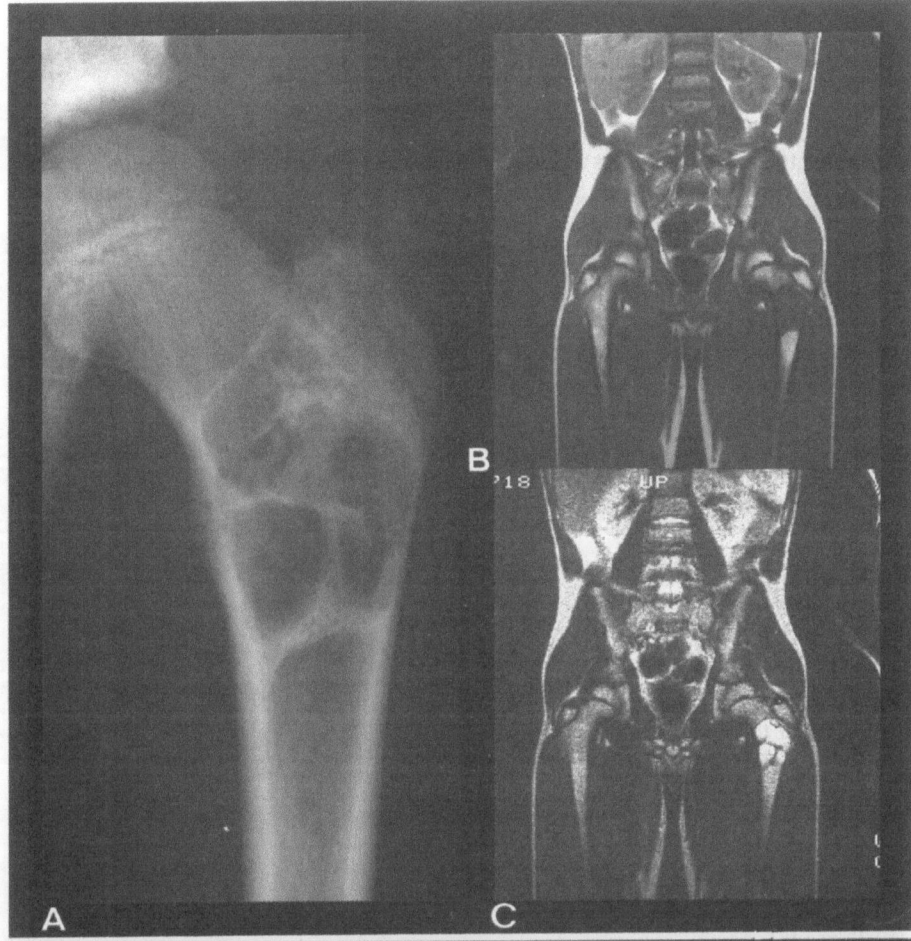

Fig. 8.1., K.R., 12 year-old male.

8.1.a. CR of the left femur.
Multilobulated, radiolucent lesion at
the proximal third of the left femur.
Minimal expansion of the cortex.
8.1.b. MRI of the left femur, coronal
section, T1-WI.
The multilobular aspect is clearly
demonstrated. Cortical bone is intact.
The lesion has a low SI [2]. Osseous
or fibrous septa separating tumoral
lobules generate no signal.
Transition zone is sharp and narrow.
8.1.c. MRI of the left femur, coronal
section, T2-WI.
The lesion has the highest SI [8],
septa remain without signal.
Diagnosis: Characteristics of multilobulated
juvenile cyst on all imaging modalities.

Fig. 8.2. B.J., 19 year-old male.

8.2.a. CR of the left humerus.
Multilobulated, trabeculated, radiolucent
lesion in the proximal meta-diaphysis
of the left humerus.
Broadening of the cortex is more
pronounced on the metaphyseal side
compared to the diaphyseal side. The
lesion is margined proximally by the
growth plate.
8.2.b. MRI of the left humerus, coronal
section, T1-WI.
The sharply delineated and lobulated
lesion presents with the SI [3] of
normal muscle.
8.2.c. MRI of the left humerus, transverse
section, T2-WI.
The internal trabeculae generate no
signal while the content of the lesion
has the highest SI [8].
Diagnosis: Characteristics of multilobulated
juvenile cyst on all imaging modalities.

52

CHAPTER 9

ANEURYSMAL BONE CYST

Aneurysmal bone cysts are mostly seen in adolescents and young adults
(second and third decade) and preferentially located in the metaphysis of
the long bones and in the spine. In 30% of the cases they occur in
association with other bone pathology. In contradistinction to simple bone
cysts they frequently cause symptoms such as pain, swelling and functio
laesa of the adjacent joints.
Aneurysmal bone cysts are blood filled spaces separated by fibrous septae,
delineated by endothelial cells and multinucleated giant cells.

Radiologically aneurysmal bone cysts are radiolucent lesions eccentrically
located in the metaphysis of the long bones. Cortical expansion (blow-up)
and internal trabeculation may be responsible for a "soap bubble aspect".
A calcified rim, a sclerotic border, an accompanying extraosseous mass
and fluid levels on CT are incidental findings.

On MRI, aneurysmal bone cysts are less homogeneous compared to simple
cysts and demonstrate a wide range of SI due to hemorrhage of different
ages. They are lobulated and completely delineated by a rim of low SI and
present the characteristic fluid-fluid levels caused by sedimentation of
blood. Diverticula-like projections arising in the walls of the larger cysts
are described (1, 2, 3, 4, 5).

References

1. Beltran JB, Simon DC, Levy M, et all. Aneurysmal bone cysts: MR imaging at
   1.5 Tesla. Radiology 1986; 158: 689-690.
2. Bloem JL, Taminiau AHM, Kieft GJ, Verbout AJ, Rozing PM.
   Kernspinresonantie-tomografie van het steun- en beenmergapparaat. Ned Tijdschr
   Geneeskd 1987; 131(30): 1311-1316.
3. Murphy WA, Totty WG. Musculoskeletal magnetic resonance imaging. Magnetic
   Resonance Annual 1986. edited by Herbert Y. Kressel. Raven Press,New York.
4. Reiser M, Rupp N, Stetter E. Erfahrungen bei der NMR-Tomographie des
   Skelettsystems. Fortschr Röntgenstr 1983; 139(4): 365-372.
5. Zimmer WD, Berquist TH, McLeod RA, Sim FH et all. Bone tumors: magnetic
   resonance imaging versus computed tomography. Radiology 1985; 155: 709-718.

COMMENT

1. Three cases of aneurysmal bone cyst are included in our series.

2. In two cases a characteristic fluid-fluid level was seen on T1-WI. Fluid-fluid level was obscured in the high SI of the lesion on T2-WI. In a third case no sagittal or transverse T1-WI were made. Consequently a potential fluid-fluid level could not be demonstrated.
In cases of cystic bone lesions T1-WI in sagittal or transverse plane are mandatory for demonstrating fluid-fluid levels.

3. Diverticula-like lesions characteristic for secondary aneurysmal bone cysts were well demonstrated in a case of non ossifying fibroma complicated by secondary aneurysmal bone cysts. Aneurysmal bone cysts had a slightly higher SI on T1-WI compared to simple bone cysts.

4. Differential diagnosis between cysts, fibrous dysplasia and some giant cell tumors is difficult on CR-CT. On MRI different SI on SE-sequences allows a more easy differentiation. Differential diagnosis between a non ossifying fibroma and an aneurysmal bone cyst was based on both morphological and SI-characteristics.

5. No contrast studies were done.

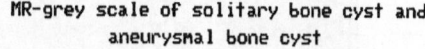

MR-grey scale of solitary bone cyst and aneurysmal bone cyst

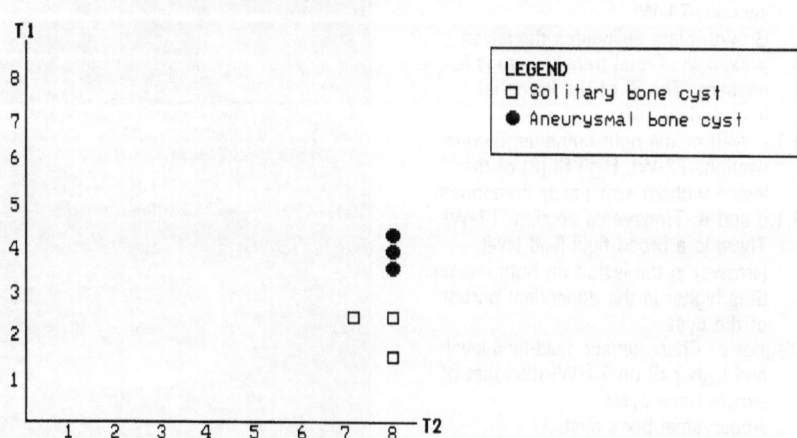

54

Fig. 9.1. M.V., 10 year-old female.

9.1.a. CR of the right humerus.
Sharply demarcated, "soap bubble"
radiolucency in the proximal
meta-diaphysis of the right humerus.
Cortical thinning and expansion.
9.1.b. MRI of the right humerus, coronal
section, T1-WI.
Growth plate delineates the lesion
proximally. Distal transition zone is
unsharp. The SI of the lesion is
intermediate [4].
9.1.c. MRI of the right humerus, coronal
section, T2-WI. High SI [8] of the
lesion without soft tissue component.
9.1.d and e. Transverse section, T1-WI.
There is a broad fluid-fluid level
(arrows) in the lesion on both images.
SI is higher in the dependent portion
of the cyst.
Diagnosis: Characteristic fluid-fluid level
and higher SI on T1-WI than that of
simple bone cysts.
Aneurysmal bone cyst.

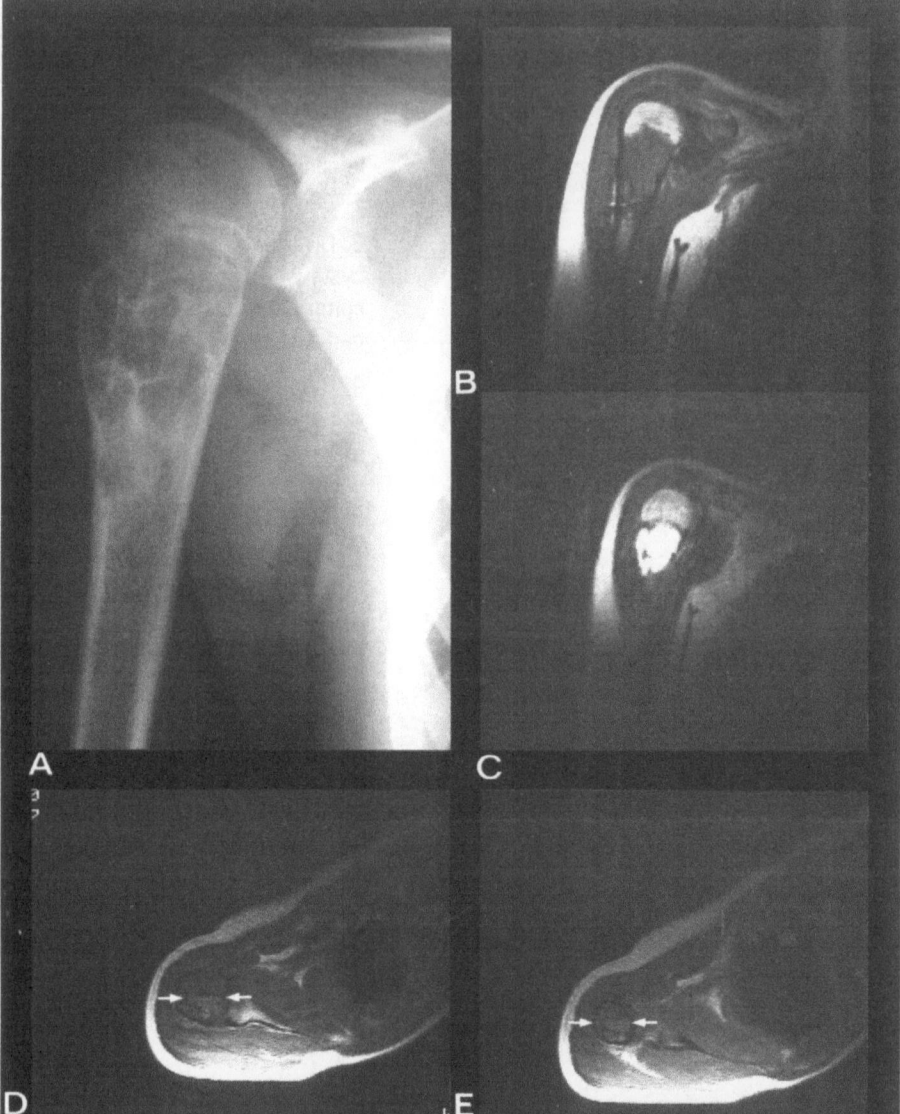

Fig. 9.2. B.M., 9 year-old male.

9.2.a. CR of the left ankle.
Radiolucent lesion at the distal third
of the right fibula. Internal trabeculation
and slight cortical expansion.
9.2.b. MRI of the left ankle, transverse
section, T1-WI.
Clearly demonstrated fluid-fluid level
(arrows). Mean SI of the lesion is
relatively high [4], SI is higher in the
dependent portion of the cyst.
9.2.c. MRI of the left ankle, transverse
section, T2-WI.
Fluid-fluid level is obscured by the
high signal of the lesion [8].
Diagnosis: Aneurysmal bone cyst with
characteristic fluid-fluid level and
increased SI on T1-WI.

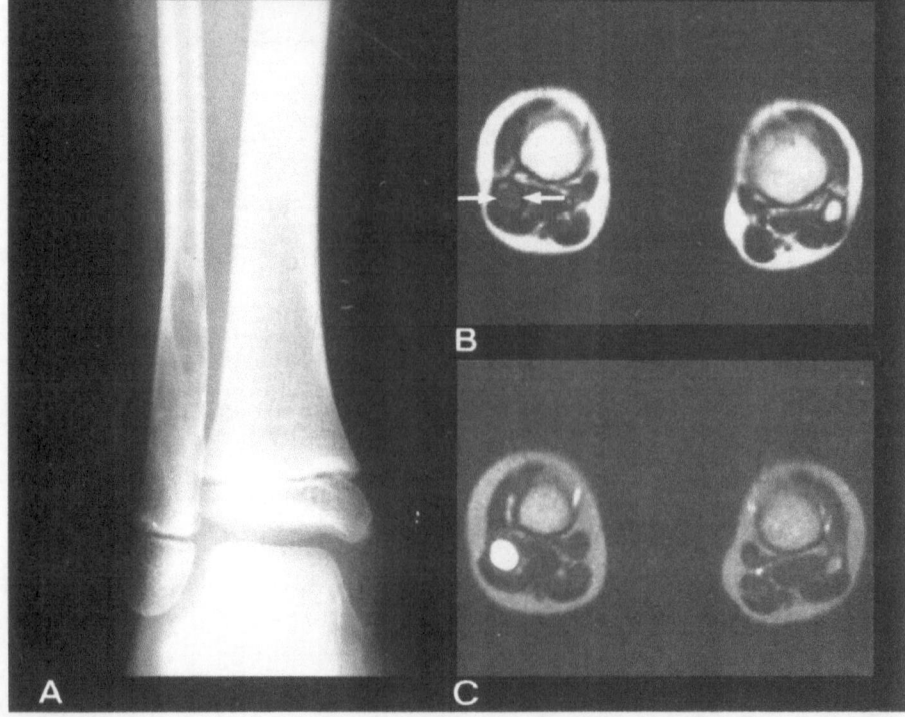

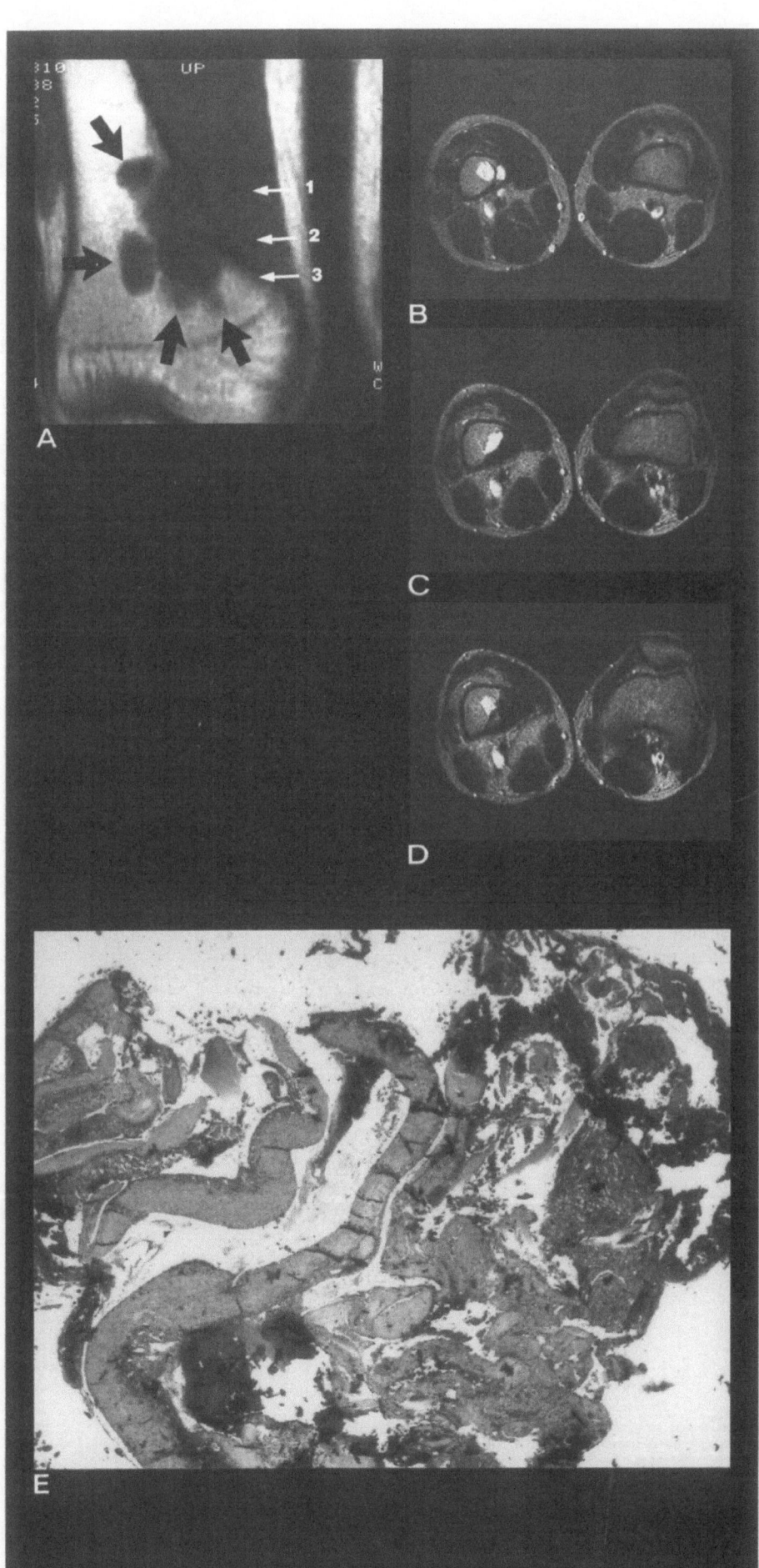

Fig. 9.3. S.M., 20 year-old male.

9.3.a. MRI of the right femur, coronal
section, T1-WI.
Multilobulated lesion, eccentrically
located at the distal meta-diaphysis
of the right femur. Slight cortical
expansion at the medial margin.
Diverticula-like projections arising in
the walls of the central lesion.
Less homogeneous, low SI [3] of the
central and peripheral components.
9.3.b, c and d. MRI of the right femur,
transverse sections, T2-WI, at the
levels indicated on the coronal image
(arrows).
The presence of two different lesions
is clearly demonstrated on these
images. A first lesion, eccentrically
located generates a poor signal [1]
while the peripheral and diverticula-like
components are of high SI [8].
9.3.e. Microphotograph (Courtesy Prof
Van Damme, KUL).
Wide vascular clefts filled with blood
and separated by loose connective
tissue septa.
Diagnosis: Pathological examination reveals
the presence of a non ossifying fibroma
and a secondary aneurysmal bone
cyst, which are both demonstrated
on MRI.

CHAPTER 10

NON OSSIFYING FIBROMA

Non ossifying fibromas are frequently seen in older children and adolescents (8 to 20 years).They are usually incidental findings. Males are slightly predilected. Histologically these brownish or orange-yellowish lesions show whorled fibrous tissue with a moderate number of giant cells, hemosiderin and aggregates of lipid-containing macrophages (lipophages).
Radiologically they consist of radiolucent, ovoid lesions, eccentrically located in the meta-diaphysis of the long bones of the lower limbs and are usually surrounded by a sclerotic rim. Long axis of the lesion (2 to 7 cm) parallels that of the limb.
No reports of MRI of non ossifying fibroma are found in the literature.

COMMENT

Although frequently encountered on CR, only one case of a large non ossifying fibroma was studied by MRI for illustrative purposes. MRI findings are not only the reflection of the predominance of the cellular component over the fibrous component but are undoubtedly influenced by the presence of hemosiderin and foam cells (lipophages). This also may explain the intermediate SI of the lesion on T1- and T2-WI and the minimal enhancement after contrast injection.

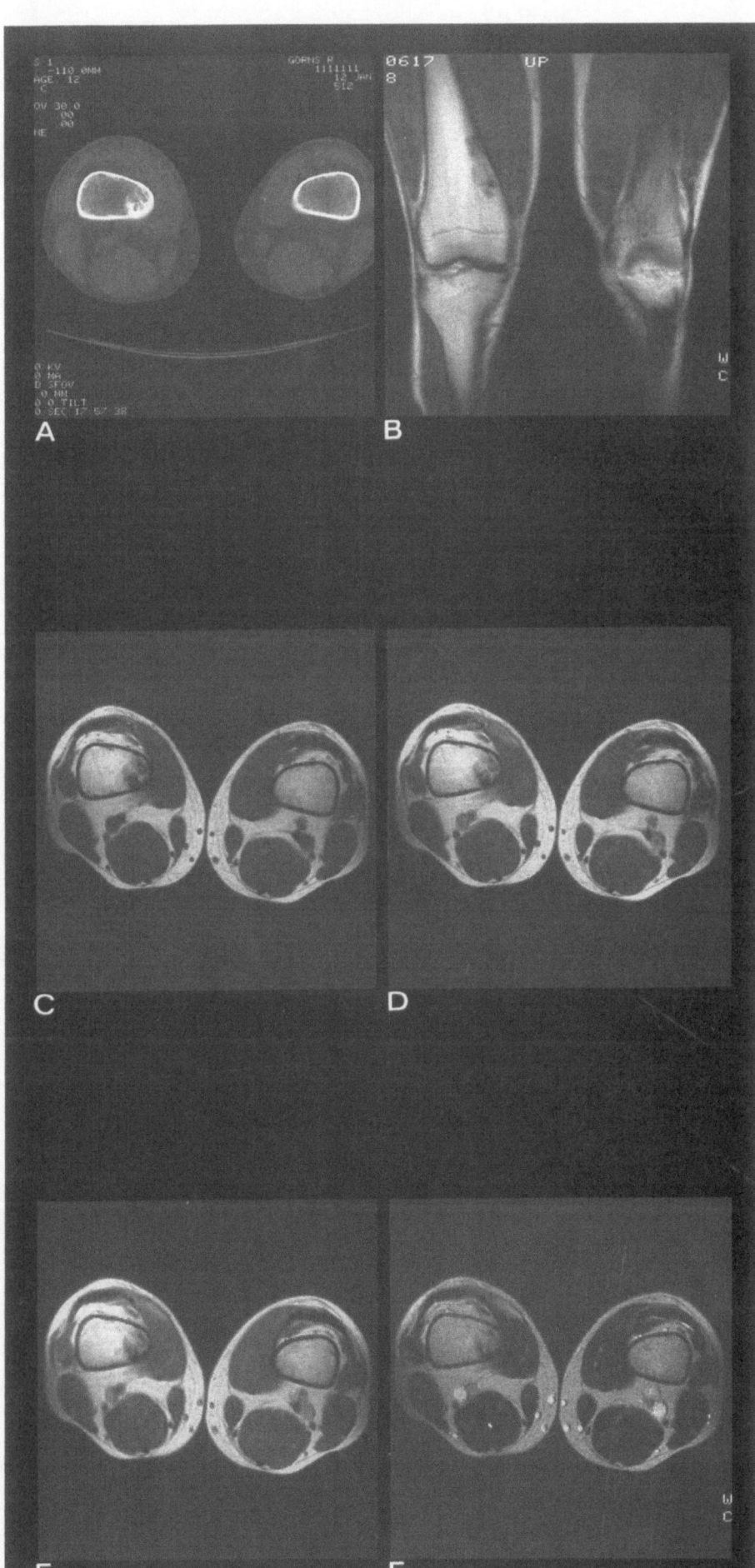

Fig. 10.1. G.R., 23 year-old male.

10.1.a. CT of the lower femoral region, soft tissue window.
Sharply demarcated lesion at the distal metaphysis of the right femur. The lesion has an eccentrical, subcortical location and a trabeculated aspect. There is no soft tissue pathology.

10.1.b. MRI, coronal section, T1-WI. Elongated, ovoid aspect of the subcortical lesion. SI is relatively high [5] with foci of decreased SI. Margins between the lesion and the adjacent medullary cavity are not well defined.

10.1.c and d. MRI transverse section, T1-WI before (c) and after (d) intravenous injection of Gd-DTPA. Only the high signal component of the lesion demonstrates a minimal enhancement.

10.1.e and f. MRI, transverse section, proton density-(e) and T2-WI (f). On T2-WI the lesion is less well demarcated from the medullary cavity. Only the low SI-foci remain visible.

Diagnosis: Non ossifying fibroma.

CHAPTER 11

EOSINOPHILIC GRANULOMA

Eosinophilic granuloma is a usually solitary bone lesion. It occurs preferentially in children and adolescents. Skull, vertebrae and long bones are most often affected. There is a slight predominance for males. Clinical signs such as fever and bone pain and neurological deficit in cases of vertebral location are reported.

The histological picture is that of a granuloma with eosinophils, lipid-containing macrophages and multinucleated giant cells.

Radiologically a well defined area of bone destruction is seen. Characteristic signs are described for location in the skull (hole-within-a-hole) and the vertebrae (vertebra plana). When located in vertebrae extraosseous extension is frequently seen, while vertebral discs are mostly preserved.

In a case reported by Haggstrom (1) vertebral eosinophilic granuloma has a low SI on T2-WI with markedly increased SI of a corresponding soft tissue component.

In contradistinction Reiser (2) reported a case with increased SI of the osseous component and an extremely high SI of the extraosseous component on T2-WI due to perilesional edema.

References

1. Haggstrom JA, Brown JC, Marsh PW. Eosinophilic granuloma of the spine: MR demonstration. J Comput Assist Tomogr 1988; 12: 344-345.
2. Reiser M, Rupp N, Stetter E. Erfahrungen bei der NMR-Tomographie des Skelettsystems. Fortschr Röntgenstr 1983; 139(4): 365-372.

COMMENT

1. Two cases of eosinophilic granuloma were studied by MRI. The first lesion was located in the vertebral body of C V, the second in the third right rib.

2. On CR-CT both lesions presented as an area of bone destruction.

3. On MRI osseous lesions had a variable SI while soft tissue components had an invariable high SI on T2-WI.

4. No definite tissue characterization was possible both on morphological features as on SI.

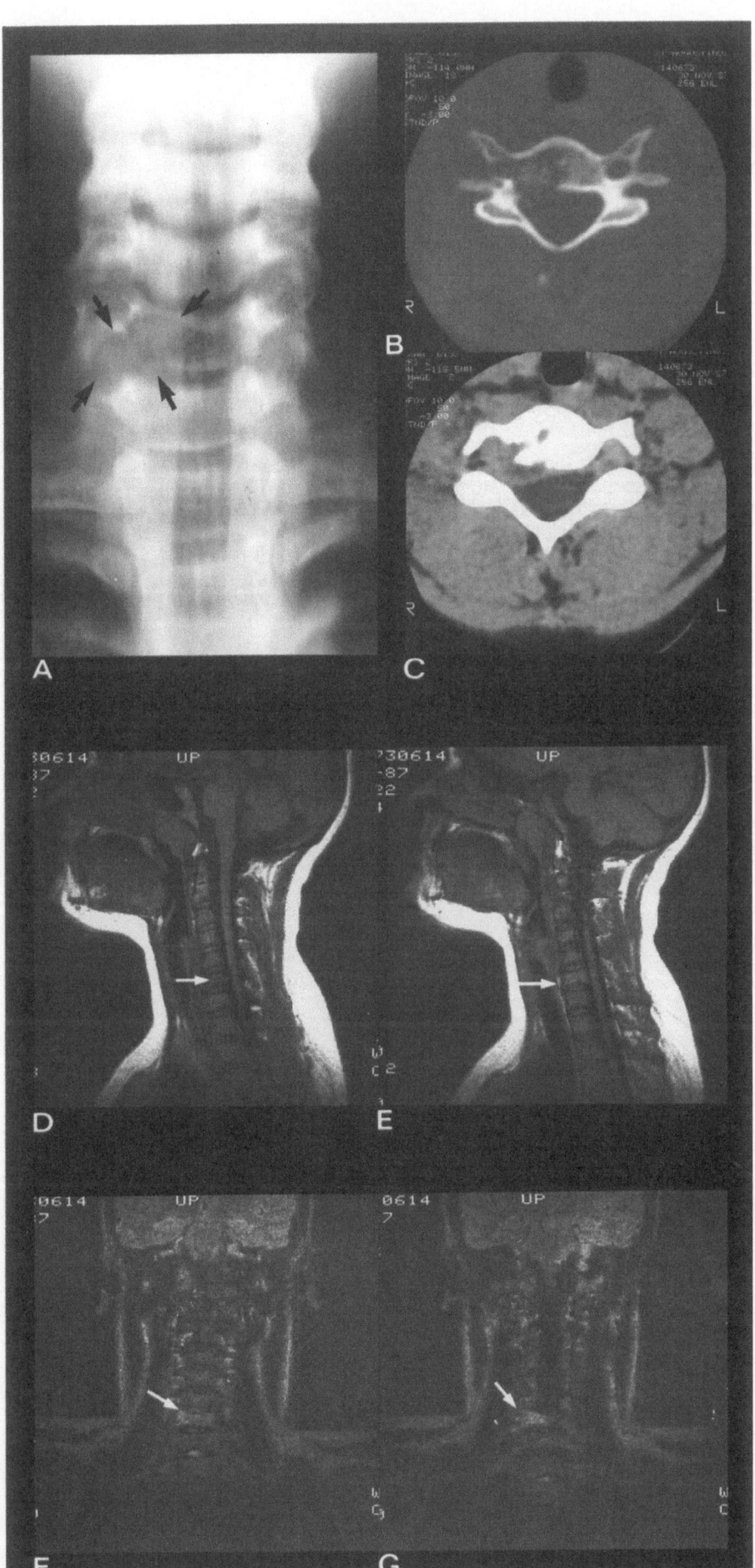

Fig. 11.1. M.M., 13 year-old female.

11.1.a. CR (tomography) of the cervical
spine.
Geographic area of bone destruction
at the right half of the body of C V
(arrows).

11.1.b. CT of C V, bone window.
Osteolytic lesion extending to the
right transverse foramen and the spinal
canal.

11.1.c. CT of C V, soft tissue window.
Extraosseous extension of the lesion
towards the spinal canal is well
demonstrated.

11.1.d and e. MRI, sagittal section, T1-WI.
The pathological vertebra has a
decreased SI on a midline sagittal
section (d) (arrows) and an increased
SI on a right parasagittal section
(e)(arrow). Enlargement of the
antero-posterior diameter with narrowing
of the anterior epidural space is best
demonstrated on the right parasagittal
section. (e)

11.1.f and g. MRI, coronal section T2-WI.
High SI [7] of both the osseous (f)
and extraosseous component (g) of
the lesion (arrows).

Diagnosis: Eosinophilic granuloma.

CHAPTER 12

FIBROUS DYSPLASIA

Fibrous dysplasia is a developmental disturbance involving proliferation
and maturation of fibroblasts and becomes clinically manifest in childhood
and adolescence, suggesting a congenital genesis. The disease is two to
three times more common in females than in males. Fibrous dysplasia may
be monostotic or polyostotic. In monostotic involvement there is a
predilection for the femur, tibia, ribs and facial bones. In cases of polyostotic
involvement there is mainly a segmental distribution i.e. one limb, trunk
bones, several vertebrae. Sometimes only one side is involved.
Clinical symptoms depend on localization and severity of involvement. Pain
and local swelling, pathologic fractures, shortening, bowing and deformity
of the bones of the lower limbs are the most common features.
Fibrous dysplasia is often associated with abnormal cutaneous pigmentation,
growth precocity, sexual precocity, hyperthyroidism, diabetes mellitus and
arteriovenous malformations.
Pathologically, fibrous dysplasia is characterized by spicules of bone and
islands of cartilage interspaced in a matrix of collagenous tissue. In the
collagenized and poorly osseous tissue areas of edematous degeneration
and cystic softening may fuse to larger cysts.
The radiological appearance is determined by the histological character of
the replacement tissue and the variable amount of bone present. If the
lesion is poorly ossified and contains cystic components it will have a
radiolucent and trabeculated aspect. If extensive ossification has taken
place the lesion has a ground glass appearance. If much cartilage is
interspersed through the replacement tissue the lesion will have a "cloudy"
or "smoky" aspect.
In two cases reported by Stark, SI was intermediate on T1-WI and low
or high on T2-WI (1).

Reference

1. Stark DD, Bradley WG. Magnetic resonance imaging. The C.V. Mosby Company,
St Louis, 1988: 1395-1396.

COMMENT

1. Five patients with proven fibrous dysplasia are included in our series.
(four monostotic and one polyostotic type).

2. In four cases fibrous tissue was characterized by an intermediate SI on
both SE-sequences. Consequently the lesions had a ground glass appearance
not only in CR-CT but also on MRI. Areas of cystification, islands of
cartilage and intralesional hemorrhage were responsible for the interspersed
areas of increased SI.
In the one remaining case the lesion was almost purely cystic with low SI
on T1- and high SI on T2-WI.

3. MRI-morphology and SI contribute to the differential diagnosis with
cystic and cartilaginous tumors which is difficult on CR-CT.
In a case of Paget's disease differentiation with fibrous dysplasia was
impossible on the basis of SI and morphological aspect. Absence of
enhancement and use of other pulse sequences (STIR) may be of additional
diagnostic value.

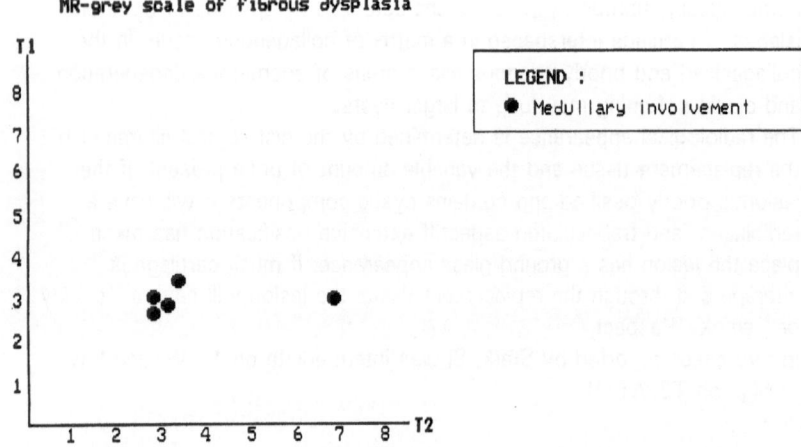

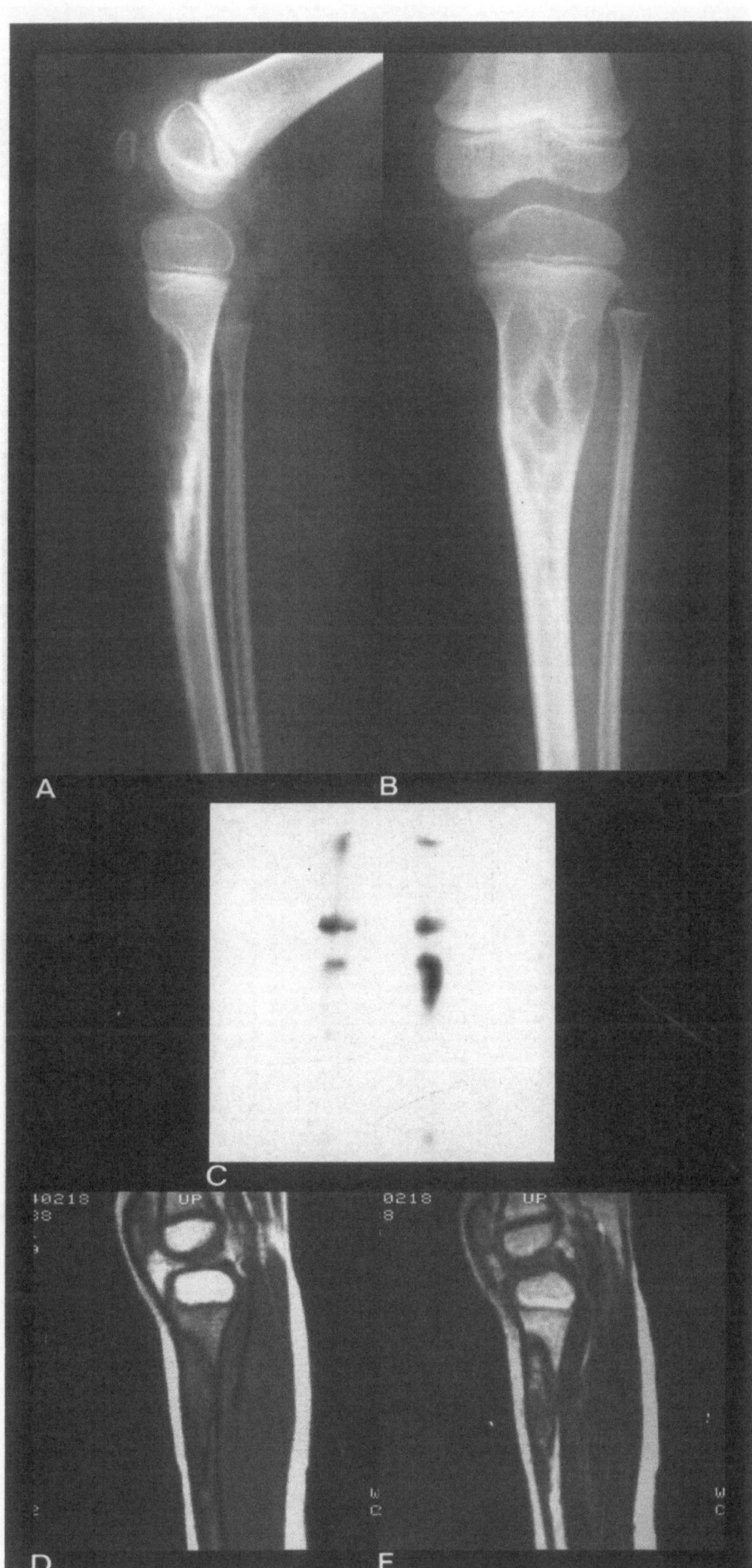

Fig. 12.1. V.T.M., 4 year-old female.

12.1.a and b. CR of the left lower leg.
Polylobular radiolucency anteriorly at
the proximal third of the left tibia.
The lesion has sharp sclerotic borders.
Cortical expansion results in an
increased latero-lateral diameter.

12.1.c. RNSC of the lower legs.
Region of tracer hyperfixation at the
proximal third of the left tibial diaphysis.

12.1.d. MRI of the left lower leg, sagittal
section T1-WI.
The lesion has an overall SI comparable
to that of normal muscle [3] with a
few areas of decreased lower SI [2].
There is a peripheral rim of low SI.
Transition zone is sharp and narrow.

12.1.e. MRI of the left lower leg, sagittal
section, T2.-WI.
Again SI of the lesion is intermediate
[4], a few areas exhibit a higher SI [5].

Diagnosis: Fibrous dysplasia (monostotic
form). Fibrous tissue with poor
ossification generates a low to
intermediate SI. Small areas of increased
SI on T2-WI are probably due to the
presence of islands of cartilage or
cystification.
The sclerotic margin is seen as a low
SI [1] rim on both SE-sequences.

64

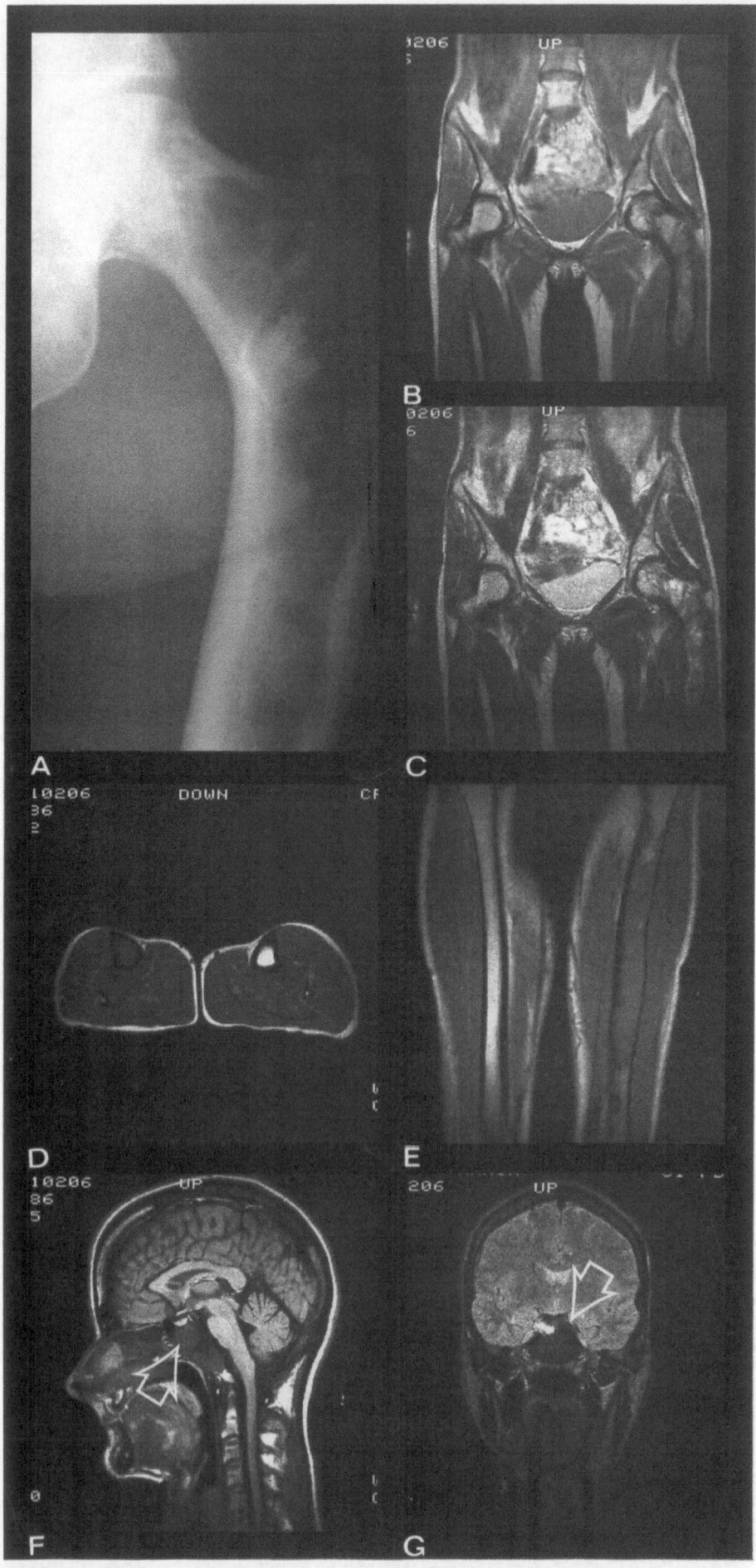

Fig. 12.2. V.D.A.M., 36 year-old female.

12.2.a. CR of the left femur.
  Enlargement of the medullary cavity,
  irregular cortical bone, epi-metaphyseal
  bowing (shepherd's crook deformity)
  and "smoky"-aspect of the left femur.
12.2.b. MRI of the upper legs, coronal
  section proton density image.
  Medullary involvement is well
  demonstrated. SI is inhomogeneous
  and slightly decreased [4] in comparison
  to adjacent normal marrow.
12.2.c. MRI, upper legs, coronal section,
  T2-WI.
  Overall SI remains intermediate [4]
  with small spots of higher SI.
12.2.d. MRI of the lower legs, transverse
  section, T1-WI.
  Cortical thinning. Medullary fat is
  replaced by tissue of intermediate SI
  [3]. Normal aspect of the adjacent
  soft tissue.
12.2.e. MRI of the lower legs, coronal
  section, T2-WI.
  Cortical thinning, enlargement of the
  medullary cavity, filled with tissue of
  intermediate SI [3].
12.2.f. MRI of the skull, sagittal section
  T1-WI.
  Lobulated mass at the level of the
  sphenoidal sinus and clivus. SI is
  intermediate [3] (open arrow).
12.2.g. MRI of the skull, coronal section,
  T2-WI.
  Also on T2-WI the mass presents
  with intermediate SI (open arrow).
Diagnosis: Polyostotic type of fibrous
  dysplasia with endocrinopathies (Mc
  Cune-Albright's syndrome).

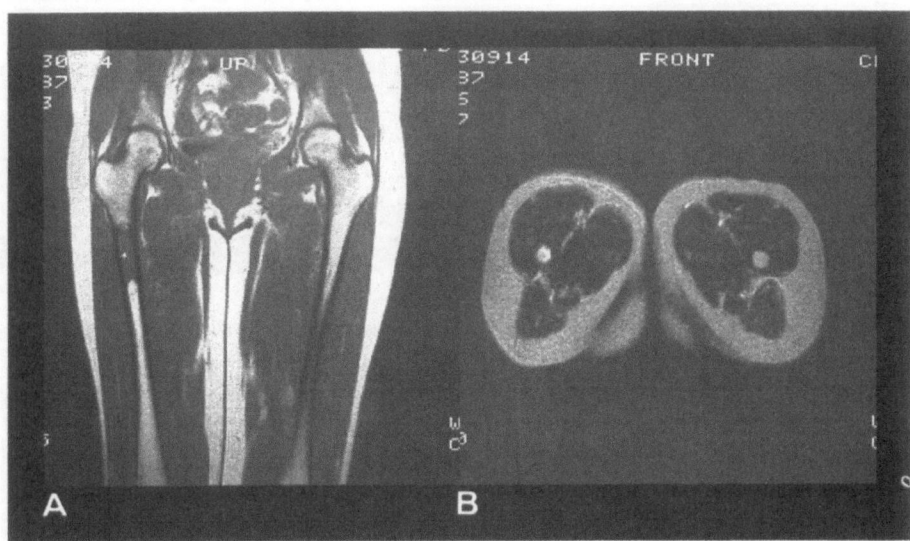

Fig. 12.3. G.F., 34 year-old female.

12.3.a. MRI of the upper legs, coronal
section, T1-WI.
Sharply delineated, homogeneous area
of low SI at the proximal third of the
left femoral diaphysis. Slight expansion
of the otherwise normal cortex.
12.3.b. MRI, transverse section, T2-WI.
The medullary bone has a high SI.
Normal appearance of the cortex and
adjacent soft tissue.
Diagnosis: Fibrous dysplasia (monostotic
form), biopsy proven.
The SI is probably due to extensive
intralesional cystification.

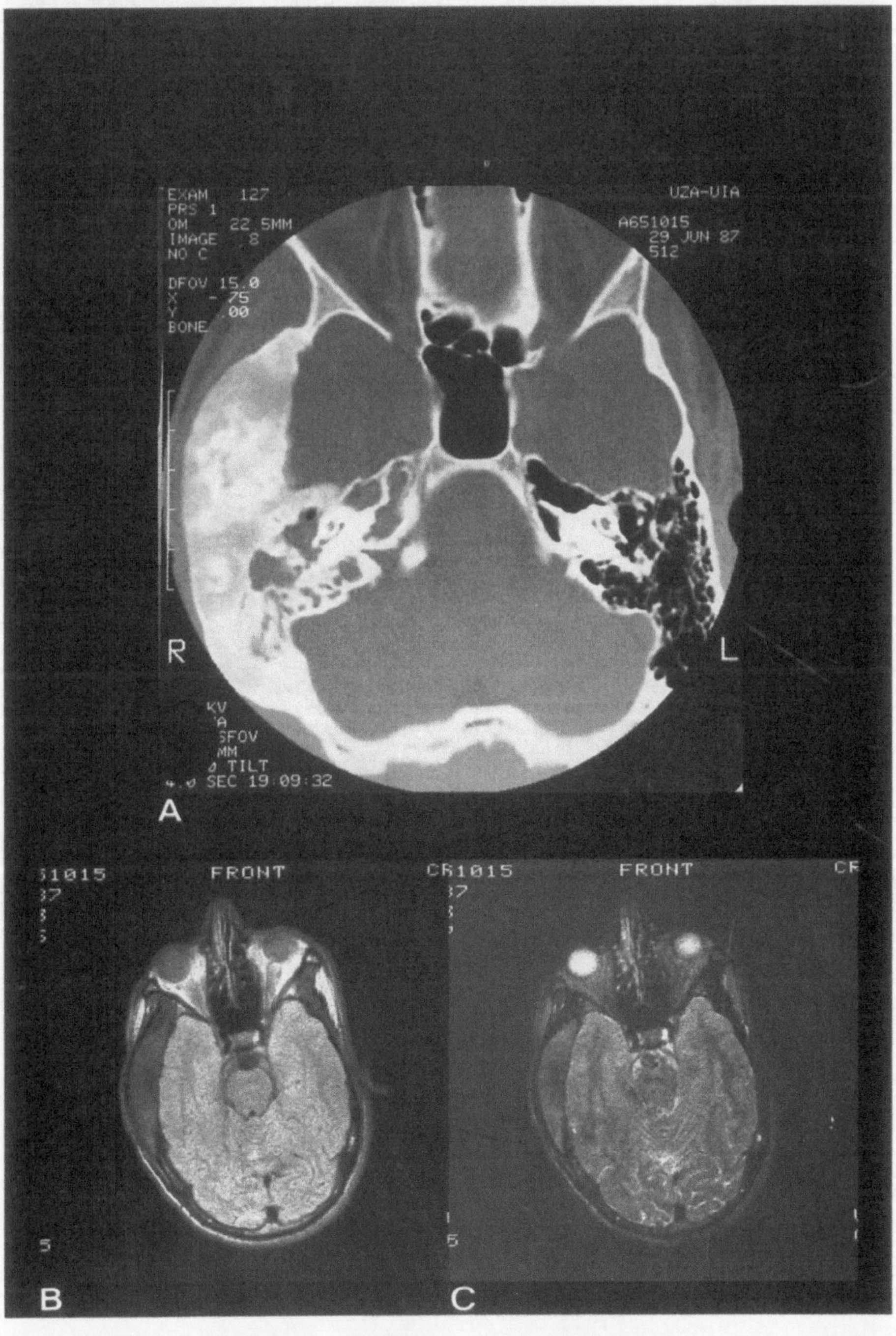

Fig. 12.4. T.M., 23 year-old male.

12.4.a. CT of the skull.
Thickening of the right temporal bone
showing an inhomogeneous, ground
glass appearance interspersed with
areas of bone density.
12.4.b and c. MRI of the skull, axial
section, proton density- (b) and T2-WI
(c).
The lesion has a crescent moon
appearance, is more sharply delineated
compared to CT and has a low to
intermediate [3][4] SI as well on
T1-(not illustrated) as on T2-WI. The
central areas of decreased SI are
presumably caused by islands of
calcified bone.
Diagnosis: Fibrous dysplasia.

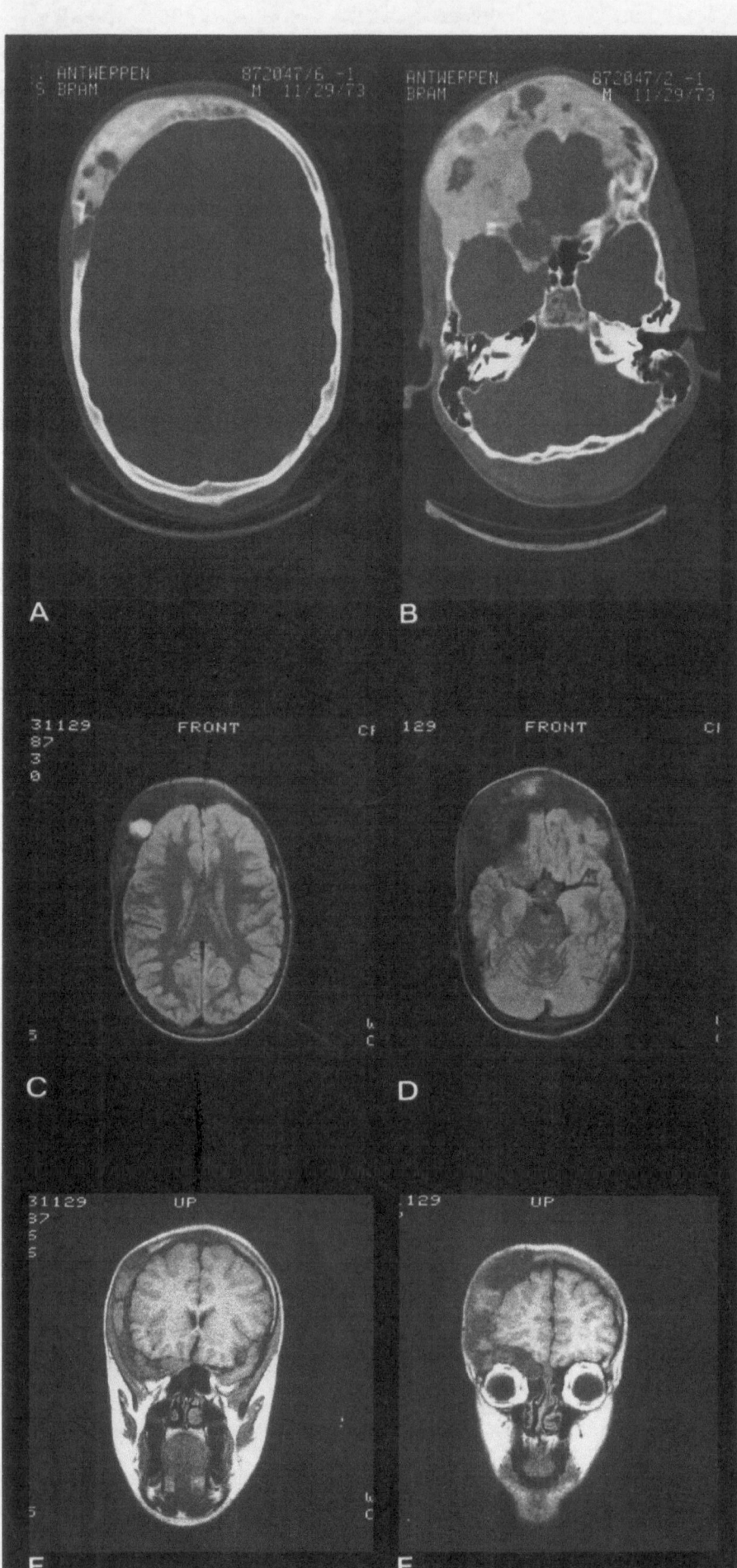

Fig. 12.5. L.B., 14 year-old male.

12.5.a and b. CT of the skull, bone window.
Irregular thickening and bossing of
the right half of the frontal bone.
The process also involves the left
half of the frontal, right ethmoidal,
sphenoidal and temporal bone. Cortical
bone has an inhomogeneous, ground
glass-appearance interspersed with
rounded-oval hypodense areas.

12.5.c and d. MRI of the skull, axial
section, proton density images.
The pathological cortical bone remains
of low SI [2]. High SI [7][8] of the
central inclusion.

12.5.e and f. MRI of the skull, coronal
section, T1-WI.
The thickened cortex has an
intermediate SI [3]. Islands of increased
SI [5] correspond to the hypodense
areas on CT.

Pathological Diagnosis: Fibrous Dysplasia.
Fibrous tissue is responsible for the
intermediate to low SI of the lesion
on both SE-sequences. The central
areas of increased SI on both sequences
probably represent a mixture of
cystification and intracystic bleeding.

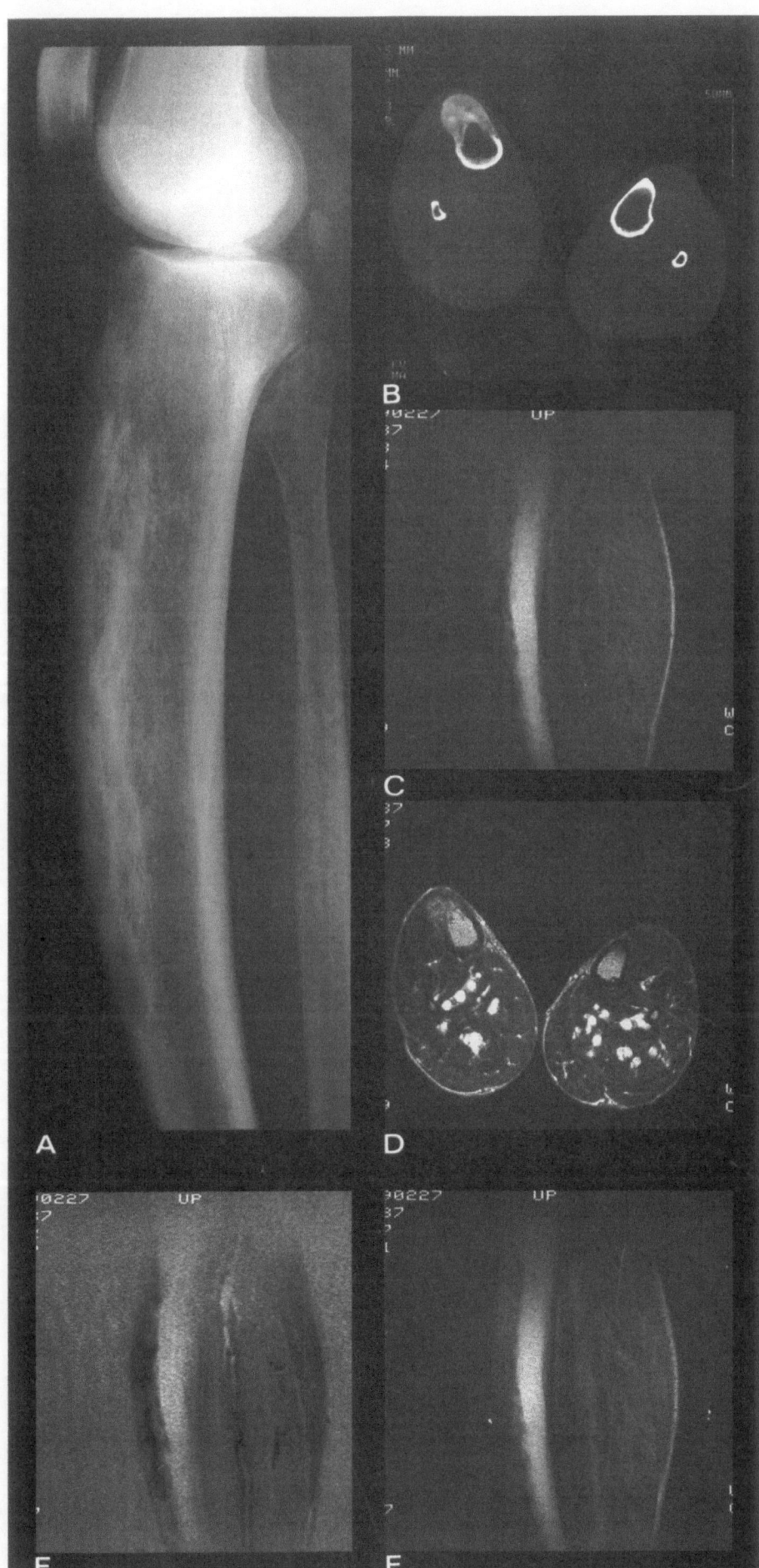

Fig. 12.6. M.P., 58 year-old male.

12.6.a. CR of the right lower leg.
Sabre sheath aspect of the left tibia, thickened lamellated cortical bone.

12.6.b. CT of the right lower leg.
Extensive thickening of the anterior cortical bone with ground glass appearance. No involvement of the medullary cavity.

12.6.c. MRI of the right lower leg, sagittal section, T1-WI.
Low to intermediate SI [2] of the anterior cortex, normal high SI of tibial bone marrow.

12.6.d. MRI of the right lower leg, transverse section, T2-WI.
Intermediate to high SI [5] of the cortical lesion. Dilatation of deep varicous veins in the lower legs.

12.6.e. MRI of the right lower leg, sagittal section, STIR.
Vermiform structures of low SI in the thickened anterior cortex. They are believed to represent flow phenomena associated with the highly vascularized bone of Paget's dysplasia.

12.6.f. MRI, sagittal section, T1-WI after injection of Gd-DTPA.
There is no enhancement of the pathological tibial cortex.

Diagnosis: Paget's disease of the tibia.

CHAPTER 13

OSTEOMYELITIS

Osteomyelitis in its different presentations may mimic tumoral conditions. Three patients with osteomyelitis are included in our study. All three patients were suspected of having a bone tumor on CR-CT, whereas both MRI and histology revealed the infectious nature of the lesion.
Staphylococcus aureus is the etiologic agent in 50% of the cases. Incidence is biphasic; osteomyelitis is mostly seen in children and in adults beyond the age of 50 years.
The disease may be hematogenous or secondary to a focus of infection. Metaphysis of long bones is a frequent localization in children, while vertebral osteomyelitis is mostly seen in adults. Pathologically it consists of bone necrosis with death of cellular constituents and disappearance of bone mass.
Initially granulocytes predominate in the inflammatory reaction but overtime they are replaced by a mononuclear infiltrate. New bone apposition originates from periosteal activation.
On MRI the lesion has a decreased SI on T1-WI and an increased SI on T2-WI. These findings are caused by inflammation and edema and due to an increased water content.
Unfortunately they lack specificity. Inflammation of adjacent soft tissue also causes an increased SI on T2, as does joint effusion and tendinitis. Cellulitis has indistinct margins while abscesses are well marginated.
In chronic osteomyelitis a rim of low SI surrounds the lesion, indicative of its benignancy (1) (2) (3) (4).
On coronal or sagittal plane examination the extent of the lesion is accurately determined allowing an optimal preoperative staging or optimal choice of biopsy site.

References

1. Beltran J, Noto AM, McGhee RB, Freedy RM, McCalla MS. Infections of the musculoskeletal system: high-field-strength MR imaging. Radiology 1987; 164: 449-454.
2. Berquist TH, Brown ML, Fitzgerald Jr RH, May GR. Magnetic resonance imaging: application in musculoskeletal infection. Magn Reson Imaging 1985; 3: 219-230.
3. Fletcher BD, Scoles PV, Nelson AD. Osteomyelitis in children: detection by magnetic resonance. Radiology 1984; 150: 57-60.
4. Zimmer WD, Berquist TH, McLeod RA, Sim FH et all. Bone tumors: magnetic resonance imaging versus computed tomography. Radiology 1985; 155: 709-718.

COMMENT

1. Three cases of osteomyelitis mimicking bone tumors are included in our series.

2. They were illustrative of different presentations of osteomyelitis in children and young adults, i.e. an acute osteomyelitis confined to the medullary cavity, a subacute osteomyelitis with cortical and soft tissue involvement and a chronic osteomyelitis with Brodie's abscess .

3. Morphological information obtained by MRI was of great value in diagnosis and differential diagnosis.
SI of the different lesions was rather aspecific but allowed in combination with morphological features a correct diagnosis in all three cases. In two cases confirmation of the exact diagnosis was facilitated by MRI-control.

4. Differentiation from Ewing's sarcoma in the first, osteosarcoma in the second and osteoid osteoma or chondroblastoma in the third case was possible.

5. No contrast studies were performed.

70

Fig. 13.1. V.D.B., 7 year-old male.

13.1.a. MRI of the lower legs, coronal
section, T1-WI.
Ill defined area of decreased SI in the
middle third of the medullary cavity
of the right tibia.
Intact aspect of the adjacent cortical
bone.
Lamellar additions of variable SI in
the adjacent periosteal region.
13.1.b. MRI of the lower legs, coronal
section, T2-WI.
The lesion in the middle third of the
diaphysis has a nearly normal SI while
proximally and distally ill defined areas
of increased SI are present. Cortical
bone remains of normal appearance
(no signal).
Periosteal reaction is demonstrated
by lamellar appositions of variable SI.
Diagnosis: Bioptically proven Staphylococcus
aureus osteomyelitis, confined to the
medullary cavity.

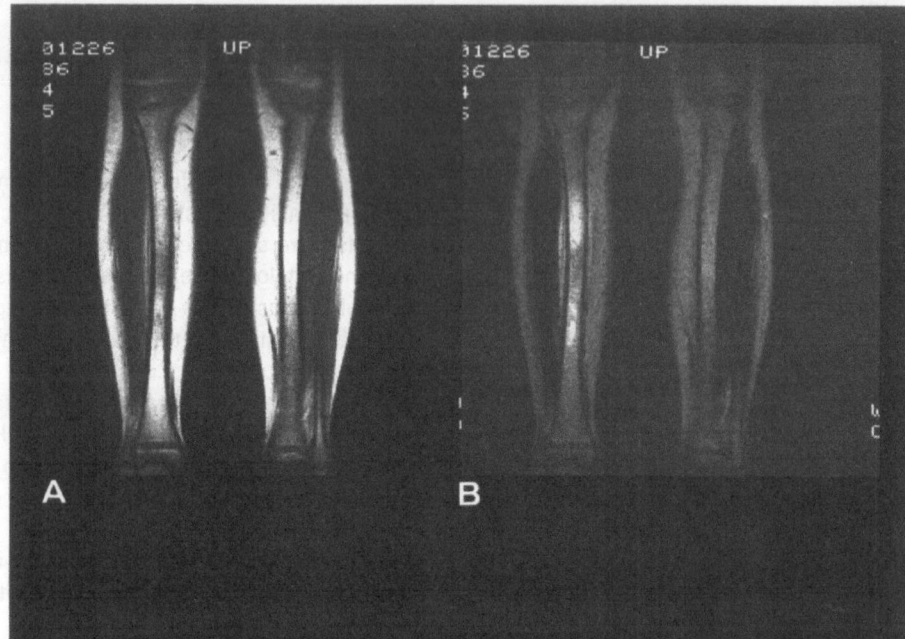

Fig. 13.2. J.P., 20 year-old female.

13.2.a and b. MRI of the upper legs,
T1-WI, before (a) and after (b) surgical
exploration.
a. Patchy decreased SI of the medullary
cavity of the right femur. Cortical
permeation is seen as areas of increased
SI. Soft tissue component of the
inflammation is seen less well on this
sequence.
b. On MRI after ten weeks of treatment
the medullary lesion is more
homogeneous and better defined.
Although cortical bone is thickened
by reactive periosteal new bone
formation, intracortical areas of
increased SI are no longer visible.
13.2.c and d. MRI of the upper legs,
T2-WI, before (a) and after (d) surgical
exploration.
c. Besides the diffuse medullary
involvement, the "dirty" aspect of
the cortical bone, inflammatory changes
in the adjacent soft tissue are seen
as areas of increased SI.
d. On MRI after ten weeks of treatment,
SI of the medullary component
decreases, cortical bone becomes
normal (without signal) and soft tissue
inflammation is no longer seen.
Moniliform structures of no signal as
well on T1-(b) as on T2-WI (d)
correspond to antibiotic pearls.
Diagnosis: This case illustrates the full
extent of a severe osteomyelitis and
the favourable evolution of the lesion
after treatment.

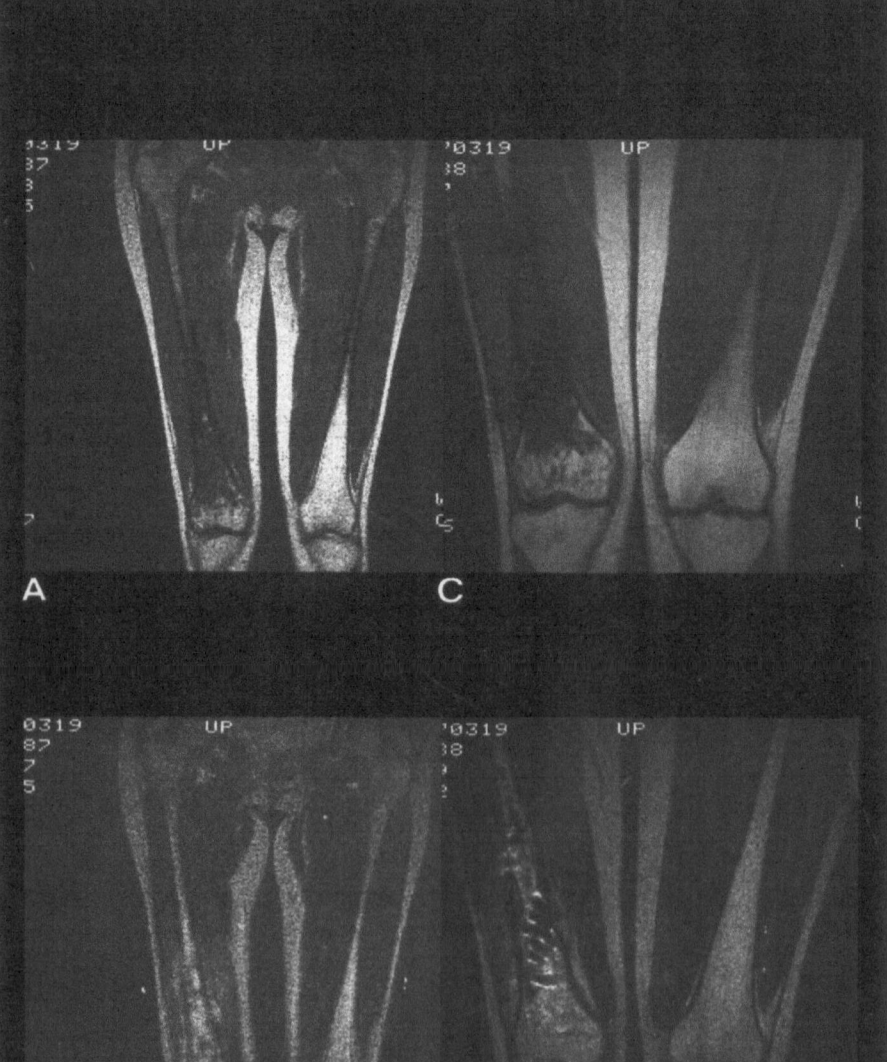

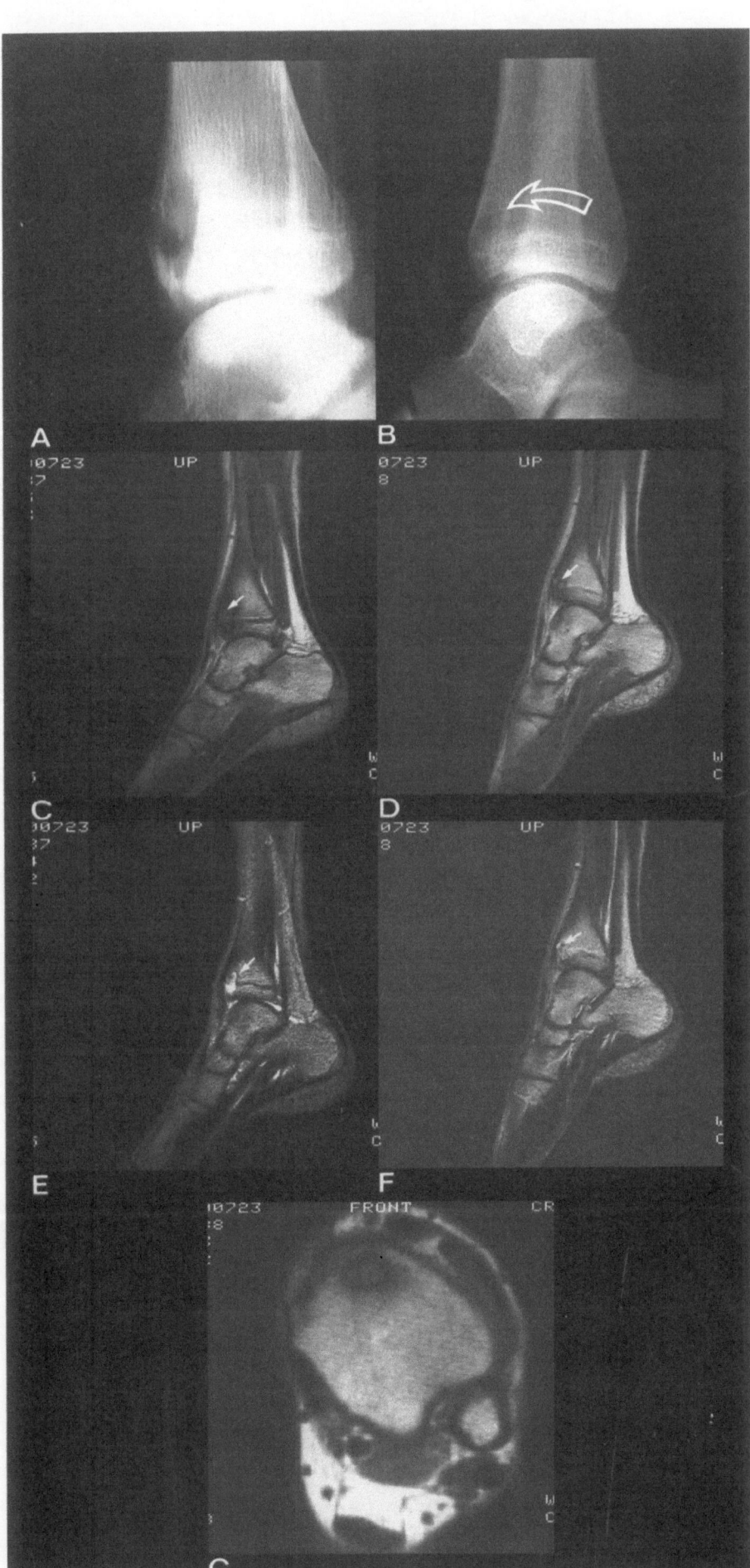

Fig. 13.3. D.B.N., 17 year-old male.

13.3.a and b. CR of the left ankle (a) and control CR after 2 months (b).
a. Sharply demarcated lytic lesion, crossing the epiphyseal plate of distal left tibia.
b. On control CR the lesion has nearly disappeared. Epiphyseal extent is no longer visible (open arrow).

13.3.c and d. MRI of the left ankle, sagittal section T1-WI (c) and control examination after 2 months (d).
c. Rhomboid area of decreased SI crossing the well visible growth plate and surrounded by a low SI rim. No evidence of joint or soft tissue involvement.
d. On control MRI the size of the lesion has definitely decreased and its SI becomes nearly equal to that of normal marrow.

13.3.e and f. MRI of the left ankle, sagittal section, T2-WI (e) and control examination after 2 months (f).
On initial MRI the lesion generates a very high signal which returns nearly to normal on control examination.

13.3.g. MRI of the left ankle, transverse section, T1-WI.
At the time of the control examination the lesion is still demonstrated in this plane.
Low intensity shell separates lesion from normal marrow.

Diagnosis: Chronic osteomyelitis (Brodie's abscess).
The initial examination already suggested the benign nature of the lesion.
MRI exactly demonstrates the residual lesion on control examination.

MALIGNANT BONE TUMORS
AND MIMICKING CONDITIONS

CHAPTER 14

OSTEOGENIC SARCOMA

Osteogenic sarcoma is a highly malignant neoplasm of bone, consisting
of a sarcomatous fibroblastic stroma in which osteoblastic activity has
induced formation of tumor osteoid and bone. After multiple myeloma,
osteosarcoma is the most common bone neoplasm. The peak incidence
is at about the age of 20 years. The tumor occurs rarely under the age
of 5 years and over the age of 40. When encountered in older patients,
osteogenic sarcoma is nearly always associated with Paget's disease or
occurs in previously irradiated bone.
Although any bone in the body may be affected, osteogenic sarcomas are
usually located in the metaphysis of long bones. Approximately 70 % of
osteosarcomas arise in the femur or tibia, mostly around the knee. When
arising in the upper extremity, the proximal end of the humerus and the
distal end of radius and ulna are favourite sites. Involvement of the vertebral
column, skull and pelvis is less common and sometimes associated with
Paget's disease.
Usually the tumor arises in the medullary bone and extends rapidly into
the medullary canal. In about 25 % of the cases, the epiphyseal cartilage
temporarily acts as a barrier, preventing tumor spread in the epiphysis.
Invasion of the joint occurs seldomly as the articular cartilage may again
slow down tumor infiltration of bone.
Penetration of the cortical bone, often associated with periosteal elevation,
is almost invariably present. The tumor may extend into the surrounding
soft tissues. In the osteolytic variant of osteosarcoma, areas of hemorrhage,
necrosis and cystic degeneration may occur within the tumor, and in this
type, infiltration into the adjacent soft tissues is more pronounced than in
the sclerosing variant.
The appearance of osteogenic sarcoma on CR-CT varies according to the
amount of tumor osteoid and bone formation. Tumors containing little
bony matrix (osteolytic variant) are seen as an ill defined lytic lesion. With
CT, areas of hemorrhage and necrosis within it can be demonstrated. In
contrast, tumors with abundant tumor bone (osteosclerotic type) are seen
as hyperdense lesions. Spicules of new bone formation, perpendicular to
the shaft cause the sunrise-appearance. Destruction of cortical bone is
very well seen with CT. Elevation of periosteum by tumor and reactive
bone development produce Codman's triangles at the junction between
normal and raised periosteum, which are well seen on CR and CT.
In the absence of tumor calcification or ossification, soft tissue involvement
cannot be assessed by CR. Although CT can demonstrate additional signs
such as tumor necrosis, suggesting extent of disease, an accurate staging
of the tumor can neither with CT be obtained. However, CT remains the
most sensitive method for demonstration of calcifications or tumor matrix
mineralization.
Staging of intraosseous extent of the tumor is not possible with CR. With
CT this extent can be roughly demonstrated, but highly precise information
is not obtained (4,5,7).
The calculation of relaxation times being not characteristic for different
tumor types, the major advantages of MRI are its highly accurate staging
capability of both intramedullary extent and soft tissue invasion by
osteosarcoma (1,2,3,4,6,7,8). As reported, MRI allows an exact evaluation
of marrow involvement, which is best seen by decreased SI of marrow
fat on T1-WI, performed along the long axis of bone (5,6,8). A sharp
delineation of the involved area would suggest a non aggressive tumor (8).
Although soft tissue calcifications or ossifications and tumor matrix
calcifications are better shown with CT, MRI is by far superior in
determination of soft tissue extent (1,4). This is best evaluated on T2-WI,

providing the greatest contrast between muscle and tumor, normal muscle being relative hypointense, soft tissue extent markedly hyperintense. As reported, inhomogeneity of this soft tissue is more pronounced in highly malignant tumors (4). In some cases the periphery of the soft tissue extent of the tumor is outlined by a low SI pseudocapsule, which is only demonstrated with MRI (8). Cortical thickening and tumoral infiltration of cortex are seen with MRI as replacement of the normally dark cortex by tissue with intermediate SI, equal to that of the invading tumor. This causes a mottled, 'dirty' aspect of the cortex and is best evaluated on axial images, both on T1- and T2-WI (8). Relationship tumor versus neurovascular structures is more easily determined with MRI than with CT, and, in addition, does not require use of contrast media. MRI is superior in detecting joint involvement by tumor (8).

References

1. Aisen AM, Martel W, Braunstein EA, McMillin KI, Philips WA, King ThF.MRI and CT evaluation of primary bone and soft tissue tumors. AJR 1986; 146: 749-756.
2. Bloem JL. Radiological staging of primary musculoskeletal tumors. Proefschrift, 's Gravenhage 1988.
3. Bloem JL, Bluemm RG, Taminiau AHM, van Oosterom T, Stolk J, Doornbos J. Magnetic resonance imaging of primary malignant bone tumors. RadioGraphics 1987; 7: 425-445.
4. Boyko OB, Cory DA, Cohen MD, Provisor A, Mirkin D, DeRosa GP. MR Imaging of osteogenic and Ewing's sarcoma. AJR 1987; 148: 17-322.
5. Gillespy Th, Manfrini M, Ruggieri P, Spanier SS, Pettersson H, Springfield DS. Staging of intraosseous extent of osteosarcoma: Correlation of preoperative CT and MR Imaging with pathologic macroslides. Radiology 1988; 167: 765-767.
6. Pettersson H, Gillespy Th, Hamlin DJ, Enneking WF, Springfield DS, Andrew ER, Spanier S, Slone R. Primary Musculoskeletal Tumors: Examination with MR Imaging compared with conventional modalities. Radiology 1987; 164: 237-241
7. Wetzel LH, Levine E, Murphey MD. A comparison of MR Imaging and CT in the evaluation of musculoskeletal masses. RadioGraphics 1987; 7: 851-874
8. Zimmer WD, Berquist ThH, McLeod RA, Sim FH, Pritchard DJ, Shives ThC, Wold LE, May GR. Bone tumors: magnetic resonance imaging versus computed tomography. Radiology 1985; 155: 709-718

COMMENT

1. Our series comprises 10 cases of osteosarcoma, examined with MRI:
2 sclerosing variants, 3 osteolytic variants, 3 chondroblastic types, 1
telangiectatic type and 1 sarcoma arising in a patient with Paget's disease.

2. Our findings in all cases did confirm the literature data i.e. MRI allowed
a better staging of both intraosseous tumor spread and soft tissue extension
compared to the other imaging techniques. Joint involvement was very
well shown on MRI, while it was difficult to assess by the other techniques
(Fig. 14.4). In the osteolytic variant and the chondroblastic type, MRI
enabled a precise definition of involved muscles, which was not evident
by the other imaging techniques.

3. A pseudocapsule around the soft tissue extent, as described by Zimmer,
was noted only in 2 of our cases (Fig. 14.2 and 14.4)(8). As there was
a disruption of it in 1 case of an aggressive type (Fig.14.4), this sign may
provide additional information about the aggressiveness of the tumor.

4. As mentioned in literature, more pronounced inhomogeneity of the
tumor and its extent was noted in the osteolytic variant than in the
sclerosing variant (Fig. 14.3)(2).

5. In our series, we noted a more pronounced T2-prolongation (higher SI
on T2-WI) in highly aggressive tumors, compared to less aggressive
neoplasms.

6. By a combination of morphological characteristics and SI itself, some
histologic variants could be predicted based on MRI-findings. For example,
this was possible in cases of chondroblastic variants of osteogenic sarcoma,
i.e. by the lobular aspect of the lesion and soft tissue extent and its very
high SI on T2-WI.

7. In five cases studies were performed after intravenous injection of
Gd-DTPA. Although this number is too small to make definite conclusions,
we believe that these contrast studies may add more specificity to the
MRI-examination, f.i. by allowing a differentiation between tumoral
involvement of soft tissues versus reactive inflammatory changes and by
specific types of enhancement for various tumors. With respect to the
latter, we noted an intense peripheral enhancement with papillary internal
borders in chondroblastic types of osteogenic sarcomas, which was
distinctive from the enhancement in the other types of osteogenic sarcoma.
However, as mentioned already, further study is needed to confirm or to
refute these preliminary observations.

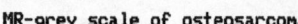

MR-grey scale of osteosarcoma

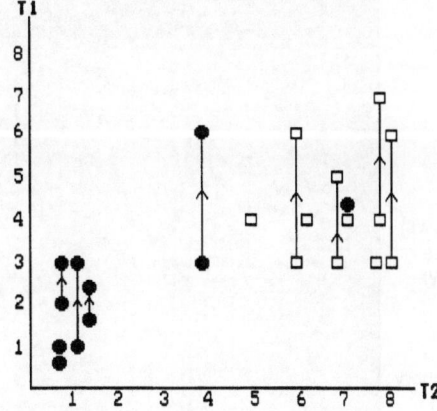

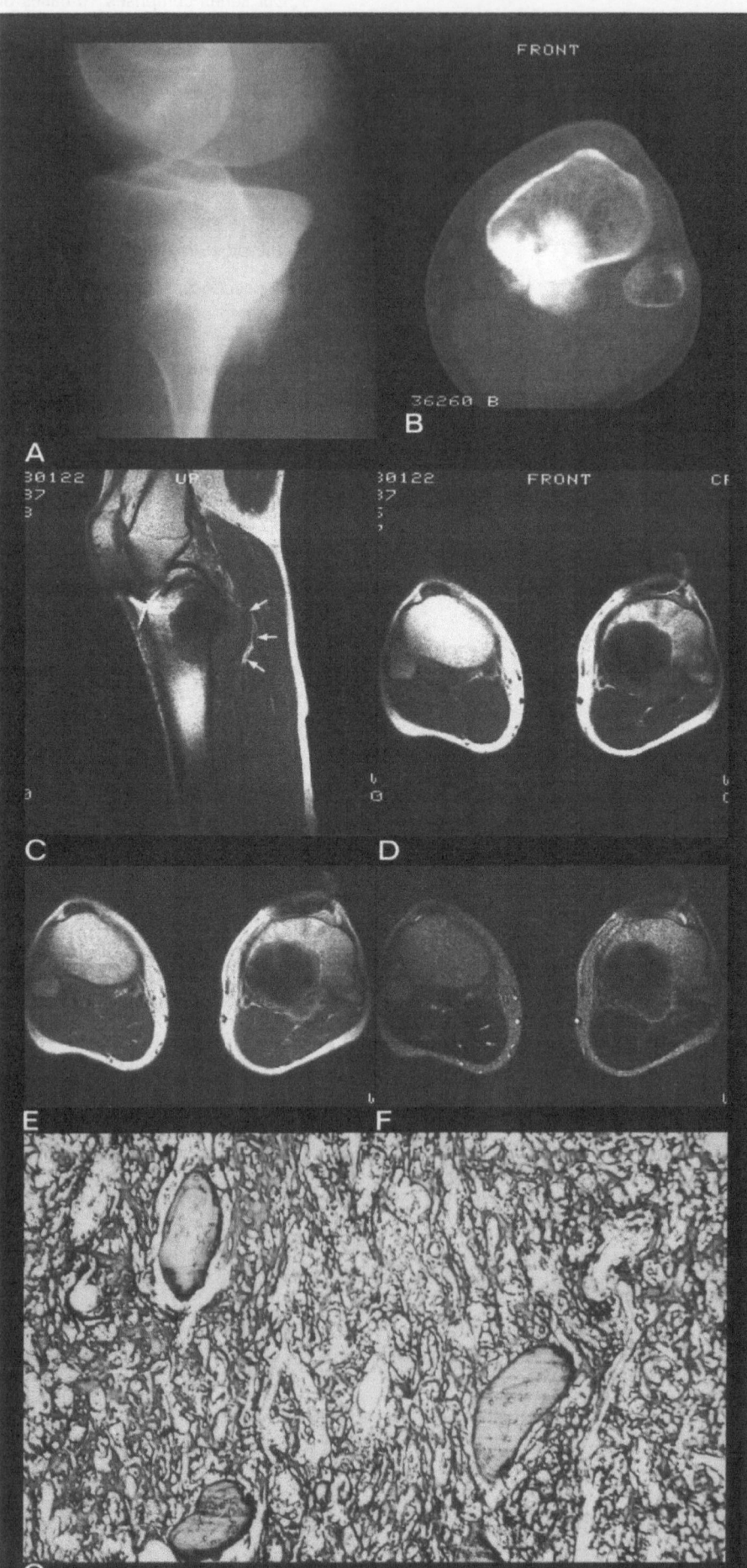

Fig. 14.1. D.K., 19 year-old male.

14.1.a. CR of the left knee.
Ill defined hyperostotic lesion at the posterior border of the proximal tibial metaphysis. Haziness of posterior tumor demarcation with spicules, indicating soft tissue involvement.

14.1.b. CT at the level of the proximal part of the tibia, bone window. Findings described on CR (Fig 14.1.a) are confirmed.
CT shows better extension of the tumor into the muscles.

14.1.c and d. MRI of the knee, sagittal section, T1-WI (c) and transverse section. T1-WI (d).
The central hyperostotic part of the tumor presents as an area of signal void [1]. Broad transition zone with intermediate SI [4] at the periphery of the lesion. Extraosseous extent into the muscles is clearly seen (arrows).

14.1.e and f. MRI of the knee, transverse section, proton density-(e) and T2-WI (f).
Again, the hyperostotic part of the tumor has an extremely low SI [1], while the transition zone at the periphery presents with intermediate SI [4]. On T2-WI, a stripe of very pronounced increase of SI is present.

14.1.g. Microphotograph of the tumor.
(Courtesy Prof Roels, RUG)
Abnormal osteoblasts, producing much osteoid tissue in pre-existing bone.

Diagnosis: well differentiated osteosarcoma, sclerosing variant.

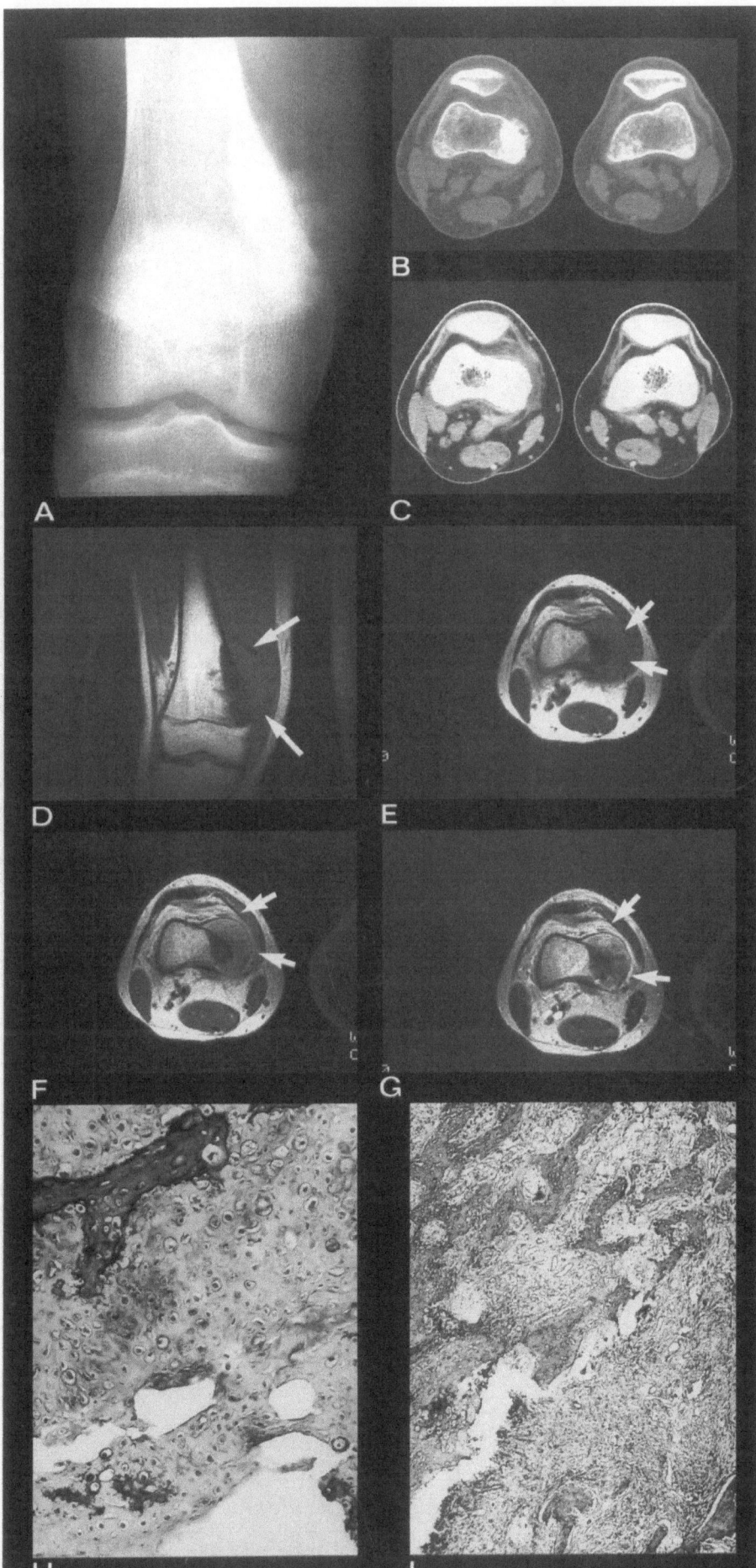

Fig.14.2. V.E.K., 17 year-old male.

14.2.a. CR of the left knee.
Irregularly demarcated hyperostotic
lesion at the medial border of the
distal metaphysis of the femur.
Tumoral new bone formation extending
into the parosteal soft tissues.

14.2.b and c. CT, section at knee level,
bone (b) and soft tissue window (c).
Confirmation of the lesion. Extent of
the hyperostotic part of the tumor
toward the medullary cavity is well
shown. Parosteal soft tissue invasion
is apparent from increased density of
the fat and from irregular thickening
of the fasciae at the medial side.

14.2.d and e. MRI at the distal part of
the femur, coronal (d) and transverse
section (e), T1-WI.
Hyperostotic part of the tumor is seen
as an area of extremely low SI [0]
[1]. Paraosseous soft tissue invasion
corresponds to the area of intermediate
SI [4], slightly higher than that of
muscle. Spicules of tumoral bone
formation are faintly seen as radiating
lines of low SI within it. Low intensity
pseudocapsule surrounding the soft
tissue component (arrow). More
peripheral involvement is suggested
by decreased SI of the fat between
the pseudocapsule and the vastus
medialis muscle.

14.2.f and g. MRI at the same level as
in fig.14.2.d and e, transverse sections,
proton density-(f) and T2-WI (g).
Hyperostotic tumor parts again appear
as areas of signal void. Foci of very
high SI [7] within the parosteal part
of the tumor are seen on T2-WI.
Invasion into the vastus medialis
corresponds to the high SI area at
the periphery of the low SI
pseudocapsule (arrows).

14.2.h and i. Microphotograph of the
tumor. (Courtesy Prof Roels, RUG).
h. Formation of abnormal cartilage by
the tumor.
i. Infiltration and destruction of
pre-exisitng bone tissue.

Diagnosis : osteosarcoma, chondroblastic
variant.

80

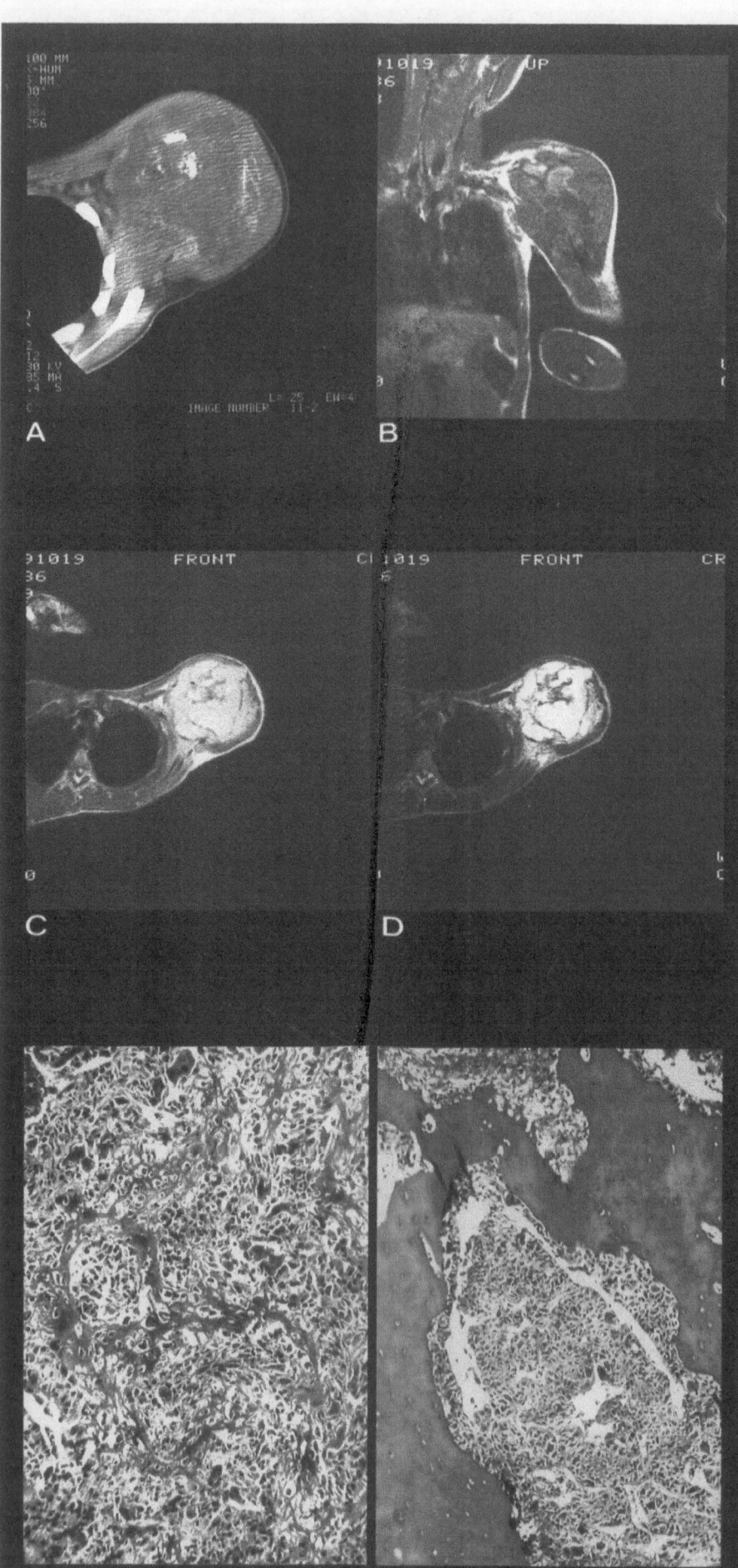

Fig.14.3. D.W.I., 17 year-old male.

14.3.a. CT at the level of the proximal
metaphysis of the humerus, soft tissue
window.
Bone destruction of the proximal part
of the humerus.
Only a few bone fragments remain.
Pronounced involvement of surrounding
tissues with large hypodense areas
of necrosis. Branched hyperdense
structure at the lateral side of the
tumor corresponds to stasis of contrast
medium in the veins.

14.3.b. MRI of the shoulder, coronal
section, T1-WI.
Clear demonstration of bone destruction.
Only a few remnants of the humeral
epiphysis and the glenoid fossa persist.
Involvement of the perihumeral muscles
seen by enlargement of them and by
inhomogeneous distribution of SI [2]
[3] in these muscles.

14.3.c and d. MRI of the shoulder,
transverse section, proton density-(c)
and T2-WI (d).
Extremely high SI [8] of the muscles,
most pronounced on T2-WI, due to
tumoral invasion and/or to reactive
edema.

14.3.e and f. Microphotograph of the
resected specimen.
e. Highly cellular osteosarcoma with
local osteoid formation.
f. Irregular border of pre-existing bone
trabeculae, due to local destruction
by tumor infiltration.

Diagnosis: osteosarcoma, osteolytic variant.

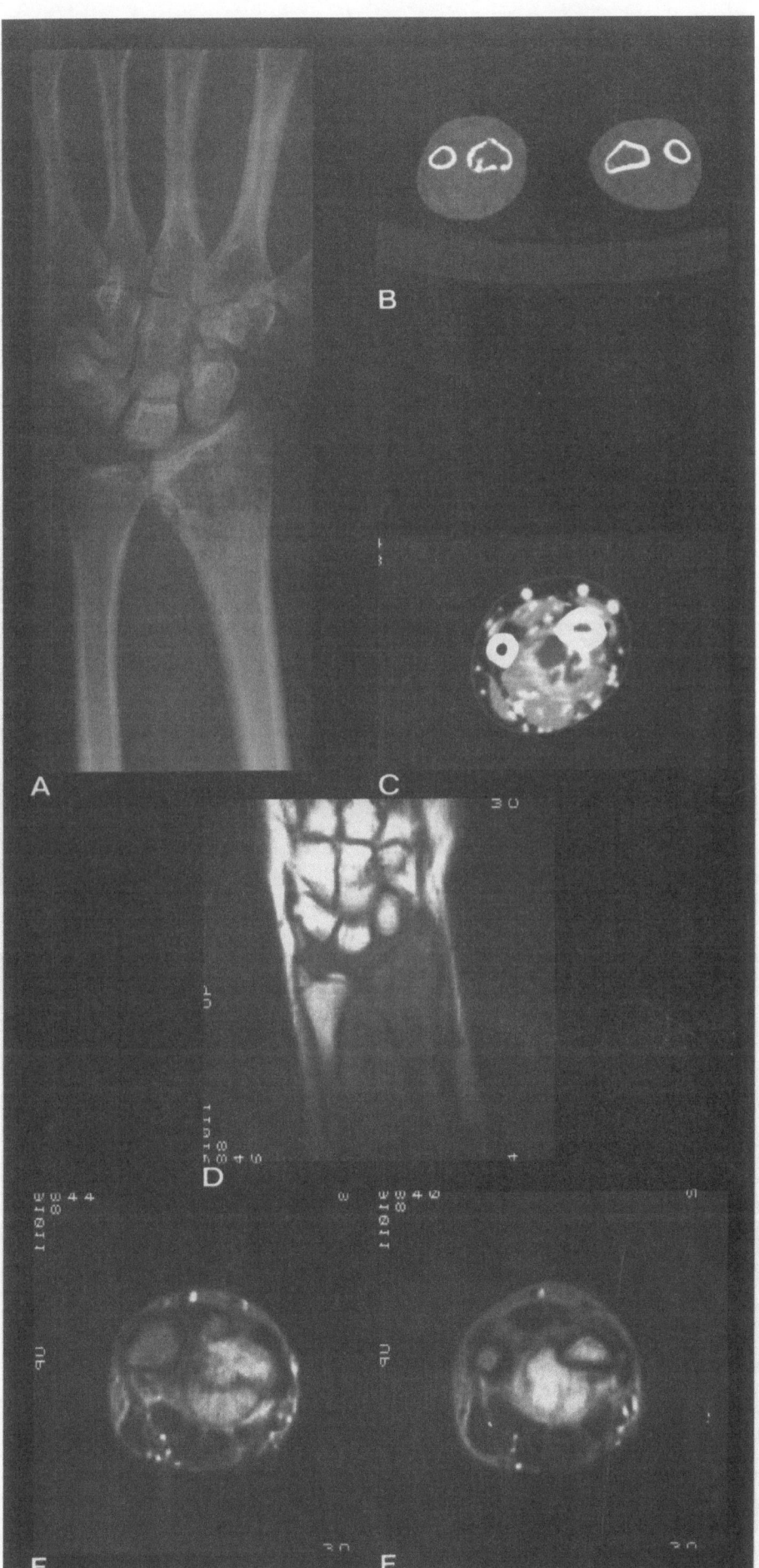

Fig.14.4. D.S.N., 19 year-old female.

14.4.a. CR of the left wrist.
Ill defined lytic lesion at the distal metaphysis of the radius. Broad transition area.
Permeative pattern of bone destruction. Permeation of the growth plate with invasion of the epiphysis.
Subtle signs of cortical permeation at the medial border of the radius at the site of the lesion.

14.4.b and c. CT at the level of the left forearm and wrist, bone window (b) and soft tissue window (c).
Cortical permeation and loss of trabecular pattern at the distal part of the radius. More proximally, extension of the tumor into the soft tissues, ventrally of the radius, is noted. The periphery of this parosteal tumor component shows pronounced enhancement after contrast injection, while the central part remains hypodense.

14.4.d. MRI of the left wrist, coronal section, T1-WI.
Inhomogeneous area of decreased SI [4] in the medullary cavity of the distal part of the radius.
Interruption of the cortical signal void with 'dirty aspect', indicating cortical destruction and permeation. Extension into the soft tissues presents as a parosteal mass of low SI [3]. Tumor spread into the radiocarpal joint is seen by enlargement of the joint space, cortical destruction of the articular surface of the radius and by presence of low SI [4] tissue within the joint.

14.4.e and f. MRI of the left wrist, transverse section at two different levels of the lesion, T2-WI.
At diaphyseal level, soft tissue component is prominent and shows a markedly increased SI [7]. No evidence for cortical permeation at this level.
At wrist level, extension into the soft tissues is clearly seen. This soft tissue component has also an increased SI [7], but is delineated by a pseudocapsule.

Diagnosis: Osteogenic sarcoma. Epiphyseal destruction, joint involvement by the tumor and presence of pseudocapsule around the parosteal tumor component are well demonstrated by MRI.

Fig. 14.5. L.D., 17 year-old female.

14.5.a. MRI of the left humerus, coronal
   section, T1-WI.
   Area of decreased SI [3] in the
   medullary cavity at the proximal third
   (meta-diaphysis) of the left humerus.
   'Dirty' aspect of the cortical bone. Ill
   defined parosteal soft tissue mass
   with increased SI [4] relative to that
   of normal muscle.
   Second area of abnormal SI [4] at the
   middle third of the medullary cavity.
   Transition zones are relatively small
   but unsharp.
   Normal appearance of the proximal
   epiphysis and growth plate.
14.5.b and c. MRI of the left humerus,
   transverse section (b) and coronal (c)
   section, T2-WI.
   b. High SI [6] of both medullary and
   soft tissue component. The proximal
   lesion has a mottled aspect and an
   intermediate SI [5].
   c. The more distal medullary lesion
   has an extremely high SI [8].
   Also high SI [6] of the parosteal soft
   tissue mass.
14.5.d. Macrophotograph of the resected
   specimen. (Courtesy Prof Van Damme,
   KUL).
   Replacement of the medullary cavity
   by abnormal tissue, which at the top
   is limited by the growth plate.
14.5.e. Microphotograph. (Courtesy Prof
   Van Damme, KUL)
   Highly vascularized and highly cellular
   osteosarcoma.
Diagnosis: Osteosarcoma, telangiectatic
   variant.
   This case illustrates well the different
   signs of a malignant bone neoplasm
   on MRI and especially well intraosseus
   tumor spread: proximally, the extent
   in the medullary cavity is stopped by
   the growth plate, while distally, tumor
   extent is separated from uninvolved
   marrow by an area of intermediate
   SI on T1-, and very high SI on T2-WI.
   The SI's of this area are consistent
   with a mixture of tumor infiltration
   and edema in the bone marrow.

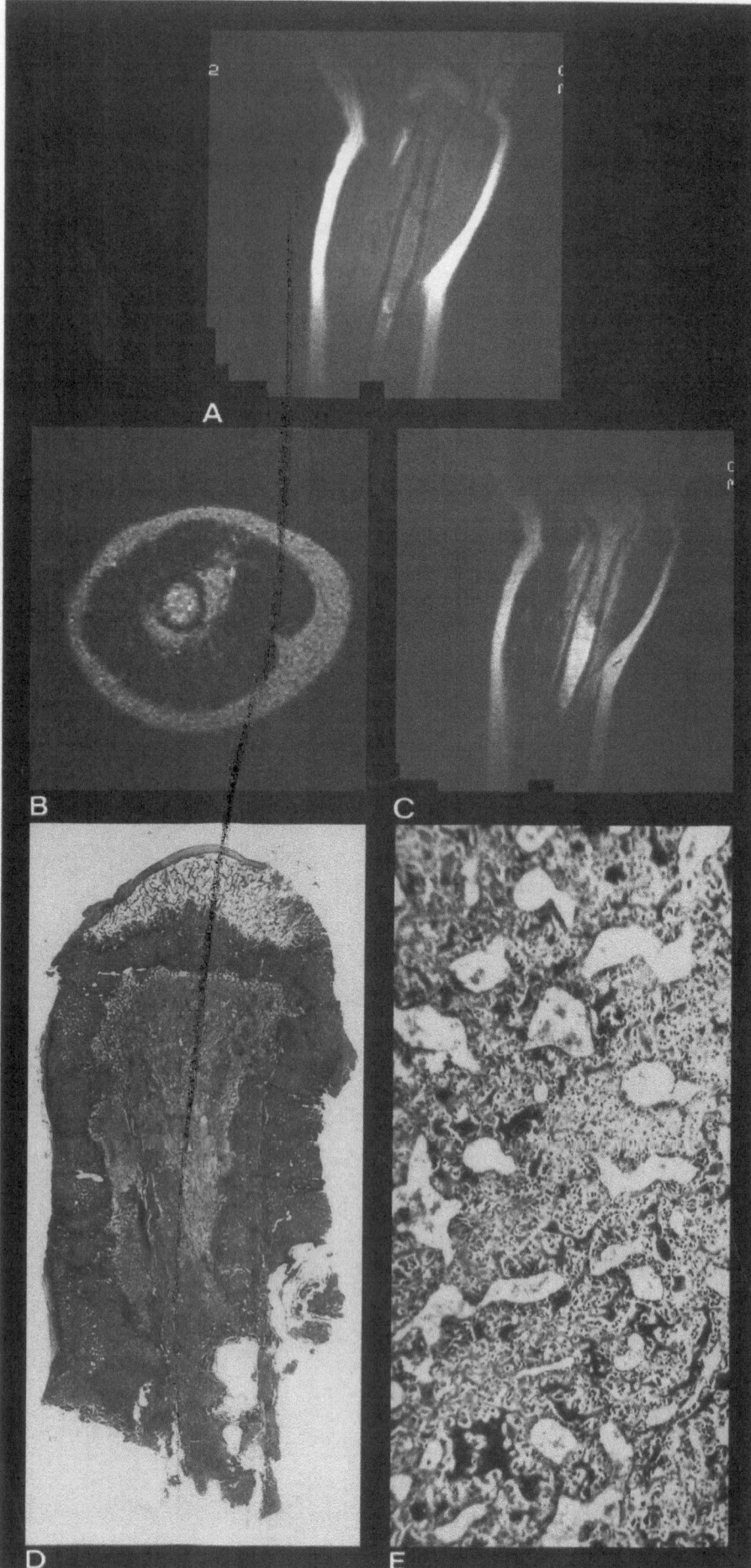

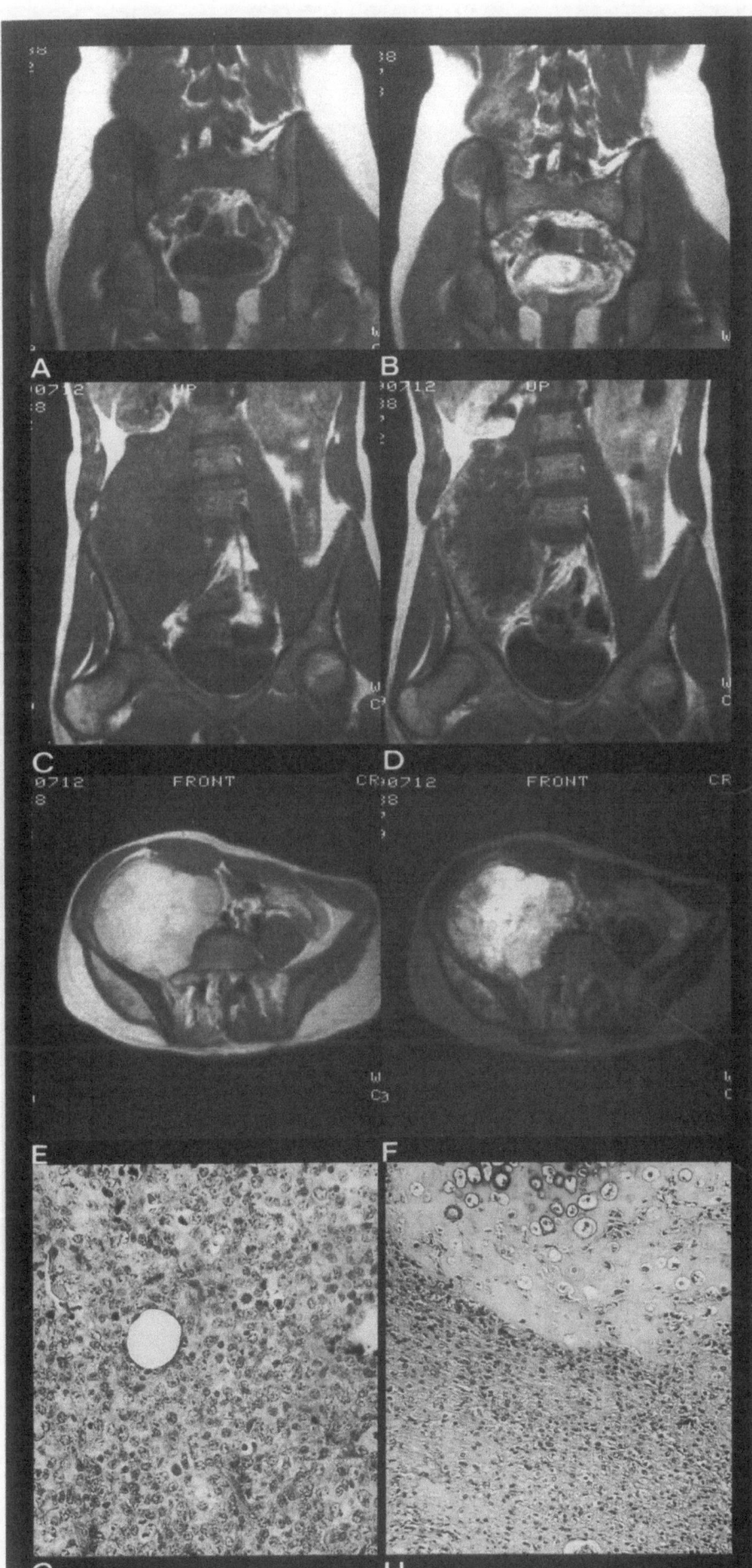

Fig.14.6. D.B.E., 18 year-old male.

14.6.a and b. MRI of the pelvis, coronal
section, T1-WI, before (a) and after
(b) intravenous injection of Gd-DTPA.
a. Area of decreased SI [1] at the
right iliac bone.
Rounded soft tissue mass lateral to
the iliac crest with an inhomogeneous,
predominantly low SI [2].
b. After contrast injection, there is
no enhancement of the osseous lesion,
while the extraosseous mass
demonstrates a peripheral, papillary
enhancement.

14.6.c and d. MRI of the pelvis, coronal
section at a more ventral level compared
to 14.6.a and b, before (c) and after
(d) injection of Gd-DTPA.
c. Huge soft tissue tumor in the right
retroperitoneal space, extending toward
the psoas muscle. The lesion has a
mottled aspect. SI is comparable to
that of normal muscle [3].
d. Peripheral papillary enhancement
of the mass.
Central area remains of low SI [2].

14.6.e and f. MRI of the pelvis, proton
density (e) and T2-WI (f).
e. Areas of low SI [2] at the right iliac
wing. High SI [7] of the intra- and
extrapelvic soft tissue masses.
f. Right iliac wing remains of low SI
[2]. The extrapelvic gluteal mass and
the peripheral zone of the intrapelvic
mass have a high SI [7]. The central
area of the intrapelvic component has
an extremely high SI [8] and a lobular
appearance.

14.6.g and h. Microphotographs of the
specimen. (Courtesy Prof Roels, RUG).
g. Osteosarcoma with chondroblastic
differentiation.
h. Highly cellular undifferentiated
osteosarcoma with many mitotic figures.

Diagnosis: Osteosarcoma, chondroblastic
variant. Lobular aspect and pattern
of contrast enhancement are findings
which are also seen in chondrosarcoma.
Hence, they may indicate the
chondromatous nature of a lesion.

84

Fig. 14.7. V.D.V.F., 22 year- old male.

14.7.a. CR of the right knee region.
Area of bone remodelling at the
proximal end of the right fibula.
Spicular, periosteal new bone formation.

14.7.b. CT of the right knee region.
Irregular thickening of the cortical
bone with spicular periosteal new
bone formation. Flecky ossification
or calcification in the medullary cavity.

14.7.c. Intraarterial DSA of the right
superficial femoral artery.
Rounded area of increased
vascularization and capillary tumoral
blush at the level of the fibular head.

14.7.d. MRI of the lower leg, coronal
section, T1-WI.
The medullary fat at the fibular head
is replaced by inhomogeneous tissue
of intermediate SI [3].
Adjacent cortical bone has a slightly
increased SI.
At the proximal third of the diaphysis,
the medullary cavity shows a definite
decrease in SI [2], while bone marrow
at the middle third of the fibular
diaphysis generates a high SI [6].
Concentrical soft tissue mass around
the fibular head with SI equal to that
of normal muscle [3].
High SI-line around the soft tissue mass.

14.7.e. MRI of the left knee, transverse
section, T2-WI.
SI at the medullary cavity remains
low [2] and cortical bone generates
no visible signal. Soft tissue mass
has a lobular, concentrical aspect and
an extremely high SI [8].

14.7.f. MRI of the left knee, coronal
section, T1-WI after intravenous
injection of Gd-DTPA.
Peripheral, ringlike enhancement of
the soft tissue lobules [5].

14.7.g. Microphotograph of the resected
specimen. (Courtesy Prof Roels, RUG).
Osteosarcoma. To the left, differentiation
into abnormal cartilage; at the right
into abnormal bone.

Diagnosis: Osteosarcoma, chondroblastic
variant.

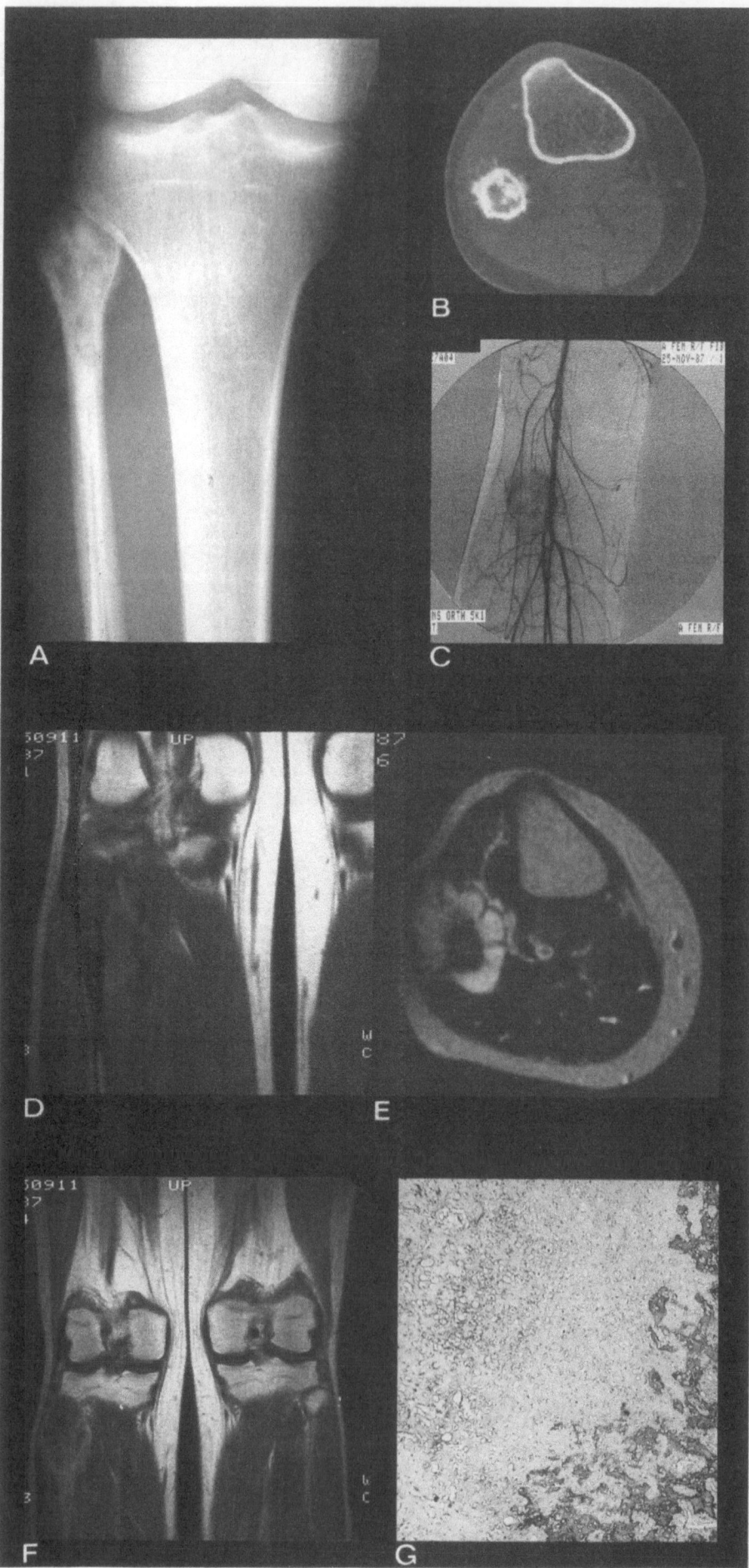

STRESS FRACTURE

Because there is an overlap in age, distribution, clinical data and even radiological appearance between stress fracture and neoplastic bone disease, MRI-characteristics of the former are described and illustrated by three cases.

Stress fractures are characterized by the absence of a well known traumatic event. They occur in normal bones due to an increased load or after a minimal trauma in patients having underlying bone diseases.

Radionuclide bone scan is extremely sensitive for detecting stress fractures, showing tracer hyperfixation, high bloodflow, increased blood pool and increased bone activity.

On conventional radiography one describes a thin cortical translucency line, a localized periosteal reaction, an endosteal thickening and a localized or diffuse bone remodelling.

On MRI only subtle cortical and medullary changes are noted at the site of the stress fracture. The lesion presents with a decreased marrow signal on T1-WI and a slightly increased SI on T2-WI. Surrounding edema is responsible for a pronounced signal raise on T2-WI [2][3]. According to Ehman these changes are observed in only half of the patients with positive bone scans (1).

References

1. Ehman RL, Berquist TH, McLeod RA. MR imaging of the musculoskeletal system: a 5-year appraisal. Radiology 1988; 166: 313-320.
2. Reither M, Kaiser W, Imschweiler E, Lindner R, Zeitler E. Bedeutung der Kernspintomographie für die Diagnostik von Knochenmarkserkrankungen im Kindesalter. Fortschr Röntgenstr 1987; 147(6): 647-653.
3. Stafford SA, Rosenthal DI, Gebhardt MC, Brady TJ, Scott JA. MRI in stress fracture. AJR 1986; 147: 553-556.

COMMENT

1. Three cases of stress fracture were studied by MRI.

2. MRI findings are consistent with literature data, i.e. patchy medullary area of decreased SI on T1-WI, and increased SI on T2-WI with high SI of the surrounding, parosteal edema on T2-WI.

3. Although in one of our cases the medullary lesion was partially obscured after contrast injection, the uniform pattern of enhancement is a useful criterion in the differentiation from neoplastic medullary involvement.

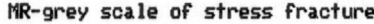

MR-grey scale of stress fracture

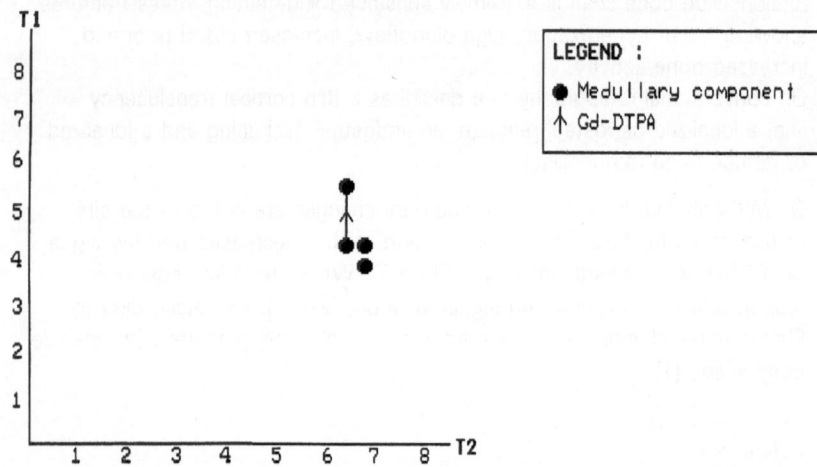

LEGEND :
● Medullary component
↑ Gd-DTPA

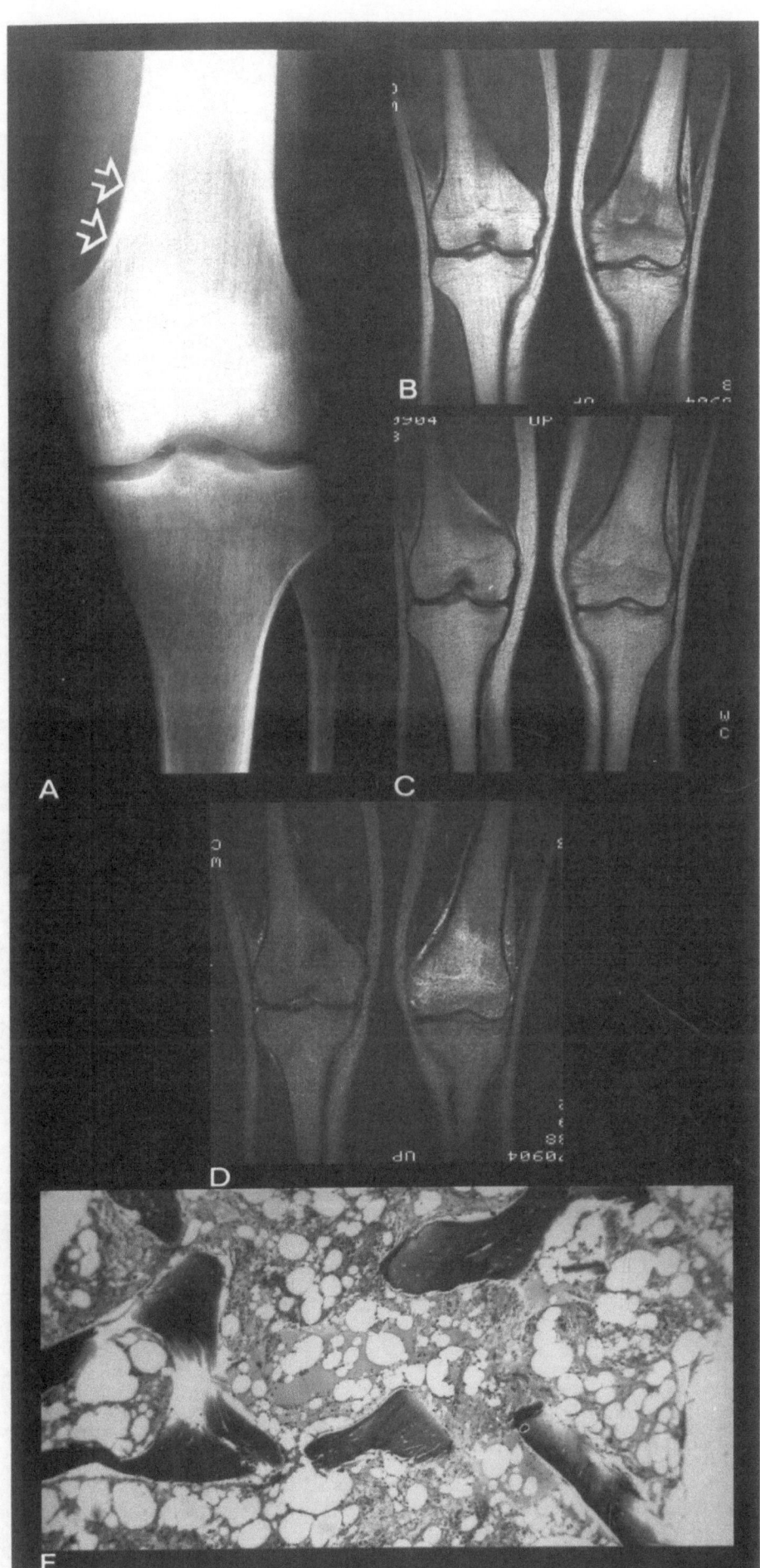

Fig. 14.8. D.S.C., 21 year-old male.

14.8.a. CR of the left knee.
Diffuse loss of bone density at the left knee region.
Discrete periosteal reaction (calcification) at the medial border of the distal metaphysis of the left femur (arrows).

14.8.b. MRI, coronal section, T1-WI.
Ill defined area of decreased SI [4] in the distal metaphysis of the left femur. Thickening of the cortical bone at the medial border. Foci of decreased SI in the parosteal fat lateral to the femur.

14.8.c. MRI, coronal section, T1-WI after injection of Gd-DTPA.
Selective enhancement of the metaphyseal lesion which becomes nearly isointense [5][6] with the adjacent bone marrow.

14.8.d. MRI, coronal section, T2-WI.
Patchy, high SI [7] of the medullary lesion.
Markedly increased SI [8] of the periosteal apposition as well on the medial as on the lateral border.

14.8.e. Microphotograph of biopsy specimen (Courtesy Dr. De Pauw, Lokeren).
Bone marrow cavities with regression of fat cells and interstitial edema.

Diagnosis: No histological evidence for infectious or neoplastic disease, despite strong suspicion of malignant bone tumor on clinical history, RNSC and CR. The findings are consistent with sequelae of a stress fracture.

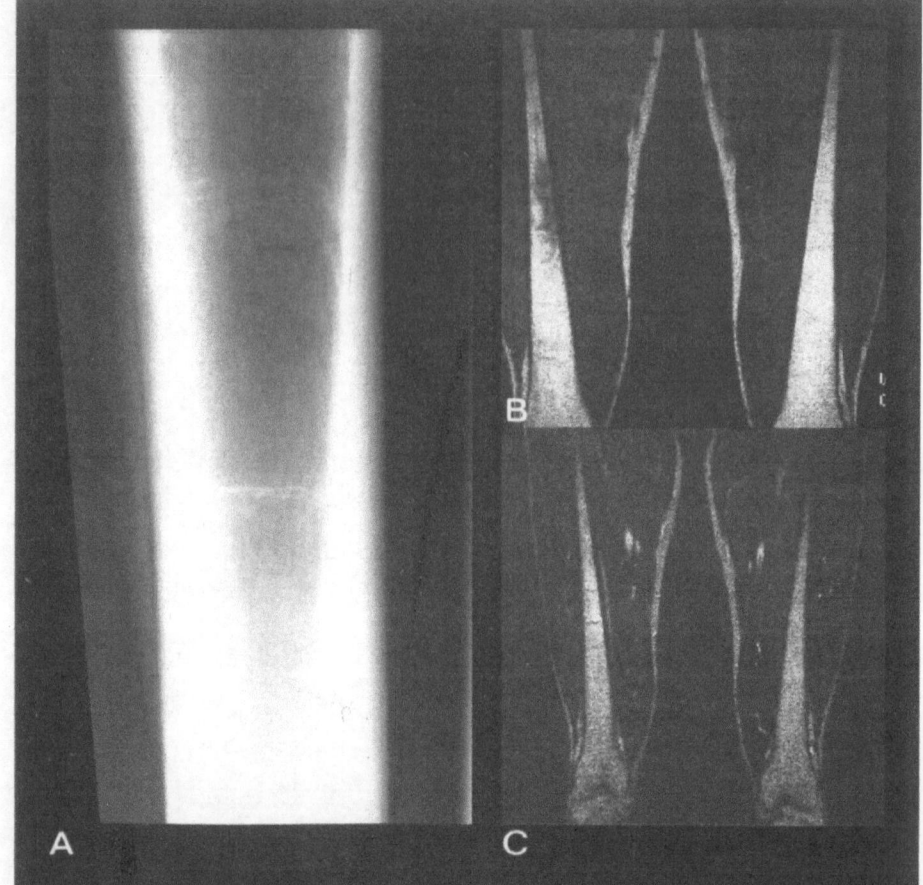

Fig. 14.9. V.D.B., 21 year-old male.

14.9.a. CR of the right femur.
Area of periosteal bone apposition
at the medial border of the femoral
diaphysis. Slight endosteal thickening.
No visible fracture. Presence of growth
lines.

14.9.b. MRI, coronal section, T1-WI.
Ill defined area of decreased SI [2] in
the medullary cavity. Cortical bone is
thickened by the periosteal apposition.

14.9.c. MRI, coronal section, T2-WI.
High SI [7] of the medullary lesion.
Low SI of the growth lines.
Parosteal high SI stripe, at the medial
border, probably due to local edema.

Diagnosis: Findings as well on CR as on
MRI are consistent with stress fracture.

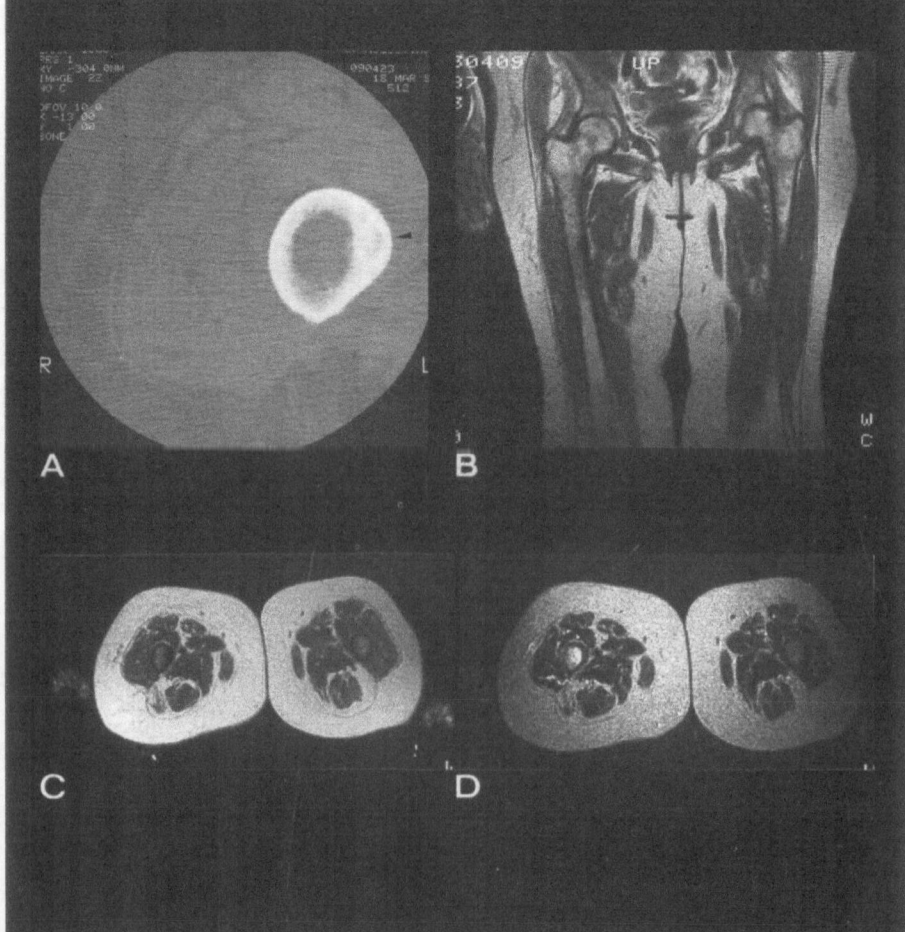

Fig. 14.10. L.E., 64 year-old female.

14.10.a. CT of the right femur, bone
window.
Cortical thickening at the medial border
of the right femur (arrowhead).

14.10.b. MRI, coronal section, T1-WI.
Patchy area of low SI in the medullary
cavity with thickening of the adjacent
cortex.

14.10.c. MRI, transverse section, T1-WI.
Confirmation of findings described in
Fig. 14.10.b.

14.10.d. MRI, transverse section, T2-WI.
High SI [7] of the medullary lesion.
Parosteal high SI stripe.

Diagnosis: Clinical evolution, CR and MRI
findings consistent with stress fracture.

CHAPTER 15

CHONDROSARCOMA

Chondrosarcoma is one of the more common malignant tumors mostly seen in adult patients, with a slight predominance for males. Preferential localizations are limb bones, scapula, ribs and pelvis. Clinically chondrosarcomas grow slowly, cause dull, local and/or intermittent pain and functional disability depending on the location.

Pathologically distinction is made between low grade and high grade chondrosarcomas. The histological and corresponding radiological characteristics of both groups have been described by Rosenthal (4). High grade tumors are characterized by a hypercellularity, a myxoid, fibrous or mixed stroma, an increased pleiomorphism with double nuclei, increased mitotic figures and bizarre cell forms.

In contrast, low grade tumors have a decreased cellular density, an abundant hyaline matrix, a limited pleiomorphism with normal mitotic activity and minimal bizarre cell forms.

Radiologically these tumors are mainly osteolytic and frequently contain amorphous calcifications. The amount of tumor calcification is thought to be inversely correlated with the malignancy grade of the chondrosarcoma (4).

The corresponding radiographic and CT-findings of high grade and low grade chondrosarcomas are summarized in Table 15.1.

TABLE 15.1. Comparison of Radiographic and CT findings in High Grade versus Low Grade chondrosarcomas

Grade	Findings
High	Faint, amorphous calcification Large noncalcified areas Concentric pattern of growth Prominent necrosis best seen on CT
Low	Dense calcification forming rings or spicules Calcification widespread or uniformly distributed Eccentric lobular growth "Pushing" margins No necrosis.

On MRI chondrosarcomas present with low SI on T1-WI. Prolongation of T1-relaxation time should be correlated with the malignancy grade, i.e. low grade tumors have an intermediate SI (moderate prolongation of T1), while high grade tumors have a low S1 (definite prolongation of T1). On T2-WI they mostly present with a high SI.

Low grade chondrosarcomas containing a hyaline cartilage matrix mostly present with a lobular aspect and a uniform, increased SI on T2-WI.

High grade chondrosarcomas containing a myxoid or cellular cartilage matrix mostly present with a inhomogeneous, intermediate SI on both SE-sequences (1) (2) (3).

90

References

1. Bloem JL. Radiological staging of primary musculoskeletal tumors. Proefschrift, s' Gravenhage, 1988.
2. Cohen EK, Kressel HY, Frank TS, Fallon M et al. Hyaline cartilage-origin bone and soft-tissue neoplasms: MR appearance and histologic correlation. Radiology 1988; 167: 477-481.
3. Petterson H, Springfield DS, Enneking WF. Radiological management of musculoskeletal tumors. Springer-Verlag. London Berlin Heidelberg New York Paris Tokio, 1987.
4. Rosenthal DI, Schiller AL, Mankin HJ. Chondrosarcoma: correlation of radiological and histological grade. Radiology 1984; 150: 21-26.

COMMENT

1. Our series comprises four cases of chondrosarcoma. A low grade chondrosarcoma (Fig.15.1) presented as a pure intraosseous lesion while in the three other cases a large soft tissue component was seen.

2. Two cases presented with the characteristic lobular appearance.

3. Medullary components had a low to intermediate SI on T1-WI and a high SI on T2-WI. The low grade chondrosarcoma had the highest SI on T1-WI.
Soft tissue components also had a low SI on T1-WI and an extremely high SI on T2-WI.

4. In one case of long bone involvement the medullary lesion was sharply demarcated, (narrow transition zone) probably due to "pushing" phenomenon (4), i.e. compression of medullary fat by tumor growth, which can also explain the increased SI of the adjacent normal fatty marrow.

5. Dirty cortex, huge soft tissue components, skip lesions, intratumoral necrosis and SI alterations in adjacent non involved muscles are characteristic signs of high grade malignancy, easily detected on MRI.

6. The statement of Rosenthal (4) that "the density of the tumor mineralization is correlated inversely with the degree of malignancy of the chondrosarcomas" was more easily demonstrated on CR-CT compared to MRI.

7. Two cases were studied after injection of Gd-DTPA. There was a moderate enhancement of the osseous component and a pronounced enhancement of the soft tissue components. In one case contrast enhancement had a ringlike-papillary pattern, in the other case a purely ringlike configuration was seen.
Central necrosis and high grade vascularization, both seen in high grade chondrosarcomas, were extremely well demonstrated on contrast studies.

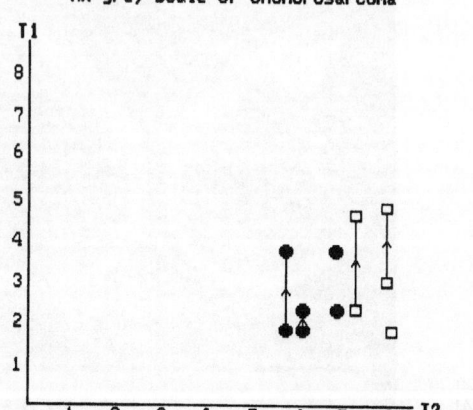

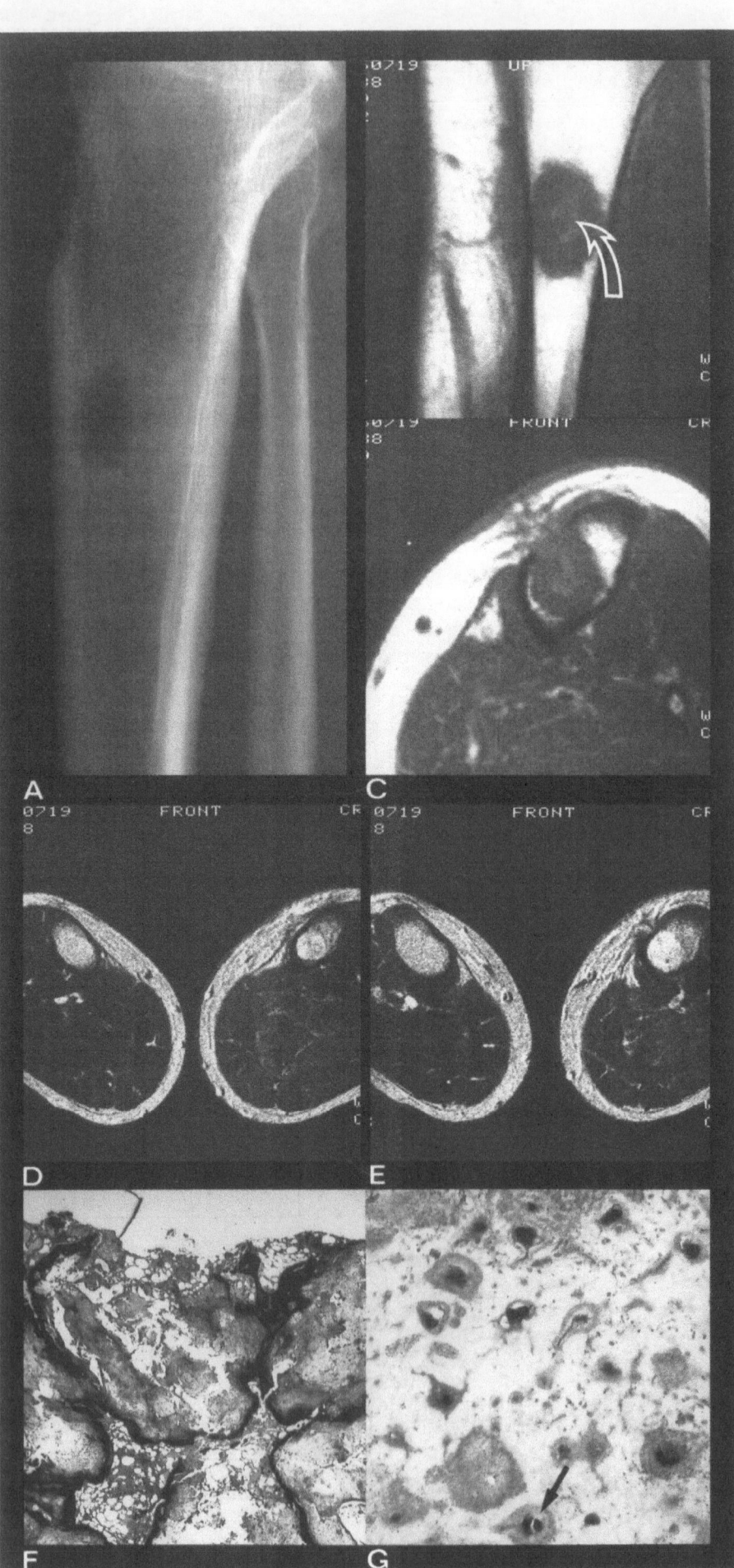

Fig. 15.1. G.J., 32 year-old male.

15.1.a. CR of the left lower leg.
Geographic, osteolytic lesion in the
tibial diaphysis.
Absence of sclerotic borders and
intralesional calcifications.

15.1.b and c. MRI, coronal (b) and
transverse (c) section, T1-WI.
Sharply demarcated medullary lesion
of homogeneous, intermediate SI [4].
The cocardelike image of higher SI
(curved open arrow) and the defect
of the anteromedial cortex are presumed
to be caused by previous biopsy.

15.1.d and e. MRI, transverse sections,
T2-WI.
High SI [7] of the medullary lesion.

15.1.f and g. Microphotographs (Courtesy
Dr.Van Hoof, Genk).
f. Low power microphotograph.
Lobulated, neoplastic cartilage nodules
surrounded by compressed connective
tissue.
g. High power microphotograph.
Individual abnormal chondrocyts with
irregular nuclei. Some cells are
binucleated (arrow).

Diagnosis: Low grade chondrosarcoma.

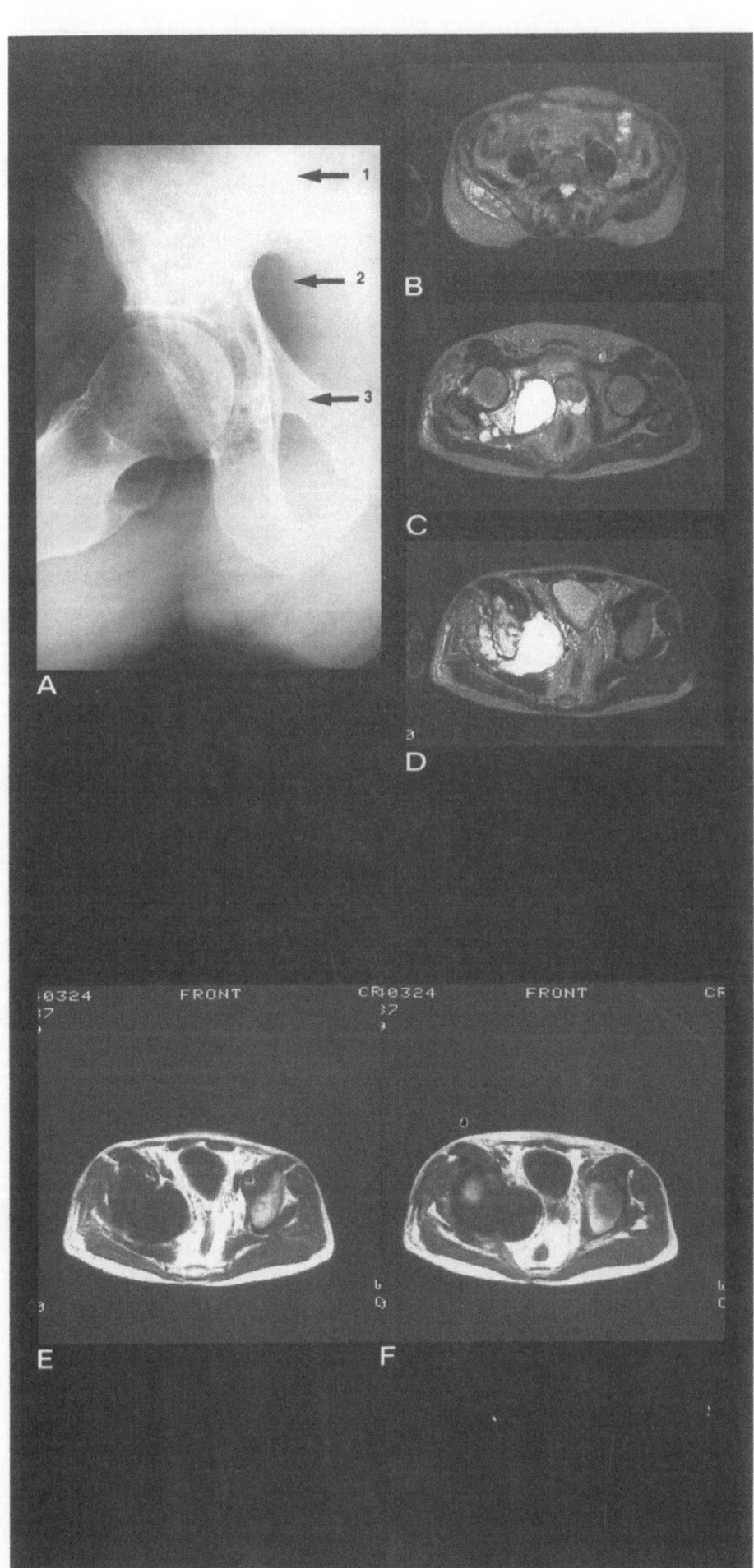

Fig. 15.2. B.J., 73 year-old male.

15.2.a. CR of the right hip region.
Faintly visible patchy appearance of
the right acetabular bone.
15.2.b, c and d. MRI, transverse sections
T2-WI at the levels indicated on the
plain film.(arrows)
b. (level 1).
Inhomogeneous, high SI of the right
gluteal muscle, without alteration of
size and shape.
c and d. (levels 2 and 3).
Lobulated soft tissue mass extending
around the acetabular bone and far
into the pelvis. A lot of secondary
lobules are seen around the central
mass. All lesions have an extremely
high SI [8]. Acetabular bone also
generates a very high SI [7].
15.2.e and f. MRI, transverse sections,
T1-WI (levels 2 and 3).
Osseous component has an intermediate
SI [3], while soft tissue mass has a
low SI [2].
Diagnosis: High grade chondrosarcoma.

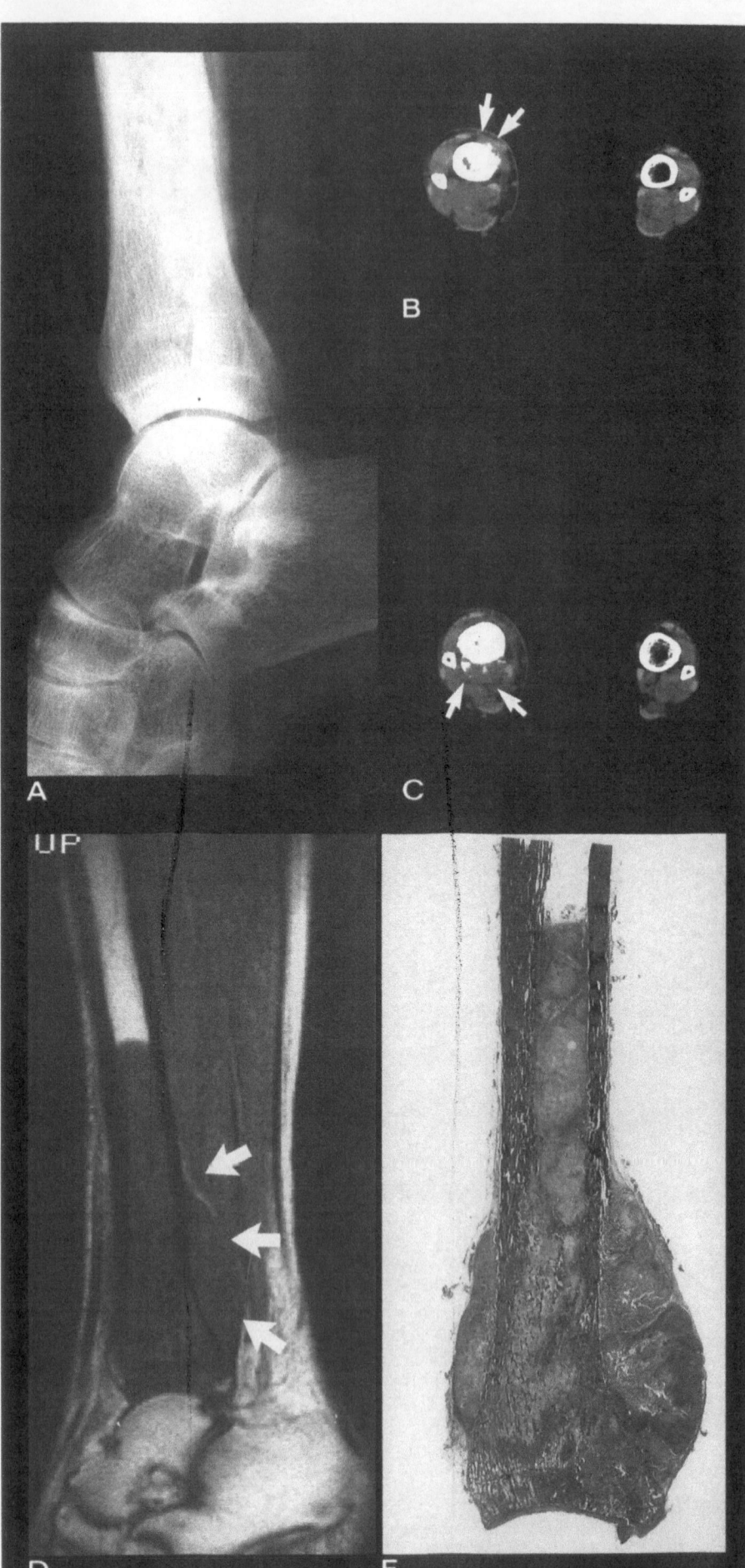

Fig. 15.3. G.H., a 45 year-old male.

15.3.a. CR of the right lower leg.
The distal third of the tibial diaphysis is diffusely hyperostotic with irregular periosteal reaction ("feu de brousse"). Transition zone is broad and ill defined.

15.3.b and c. CT scan, soft tissue window.
CT scan shows a concentric thickening of the cortex.
Irregular, amorphous endosteal and parosteal calcifications. Parosteal soft tissue component at the dorsal and anteromedial borders of the lesion (arrows).

15.3.d. MRI, sagittal section T1-WI.
The tumor and its intramedullary extent both have a low SI [3]. Note the sharp demarcation of the intramedullary tumor extension.
The parosteal soft tissue extent of the tumor posterior to the tibia, has the same SI as muscle [3], and is only seen by displacement of surrounding fat plane (arrows).

15.3.e. Macroscopic specimen, sagittal section (Courtesy Prof Van Damme, KUL). Remarkable similarity between the presence and the extension of the different tumor components compared to MRI (Fig. 15.3.d.).

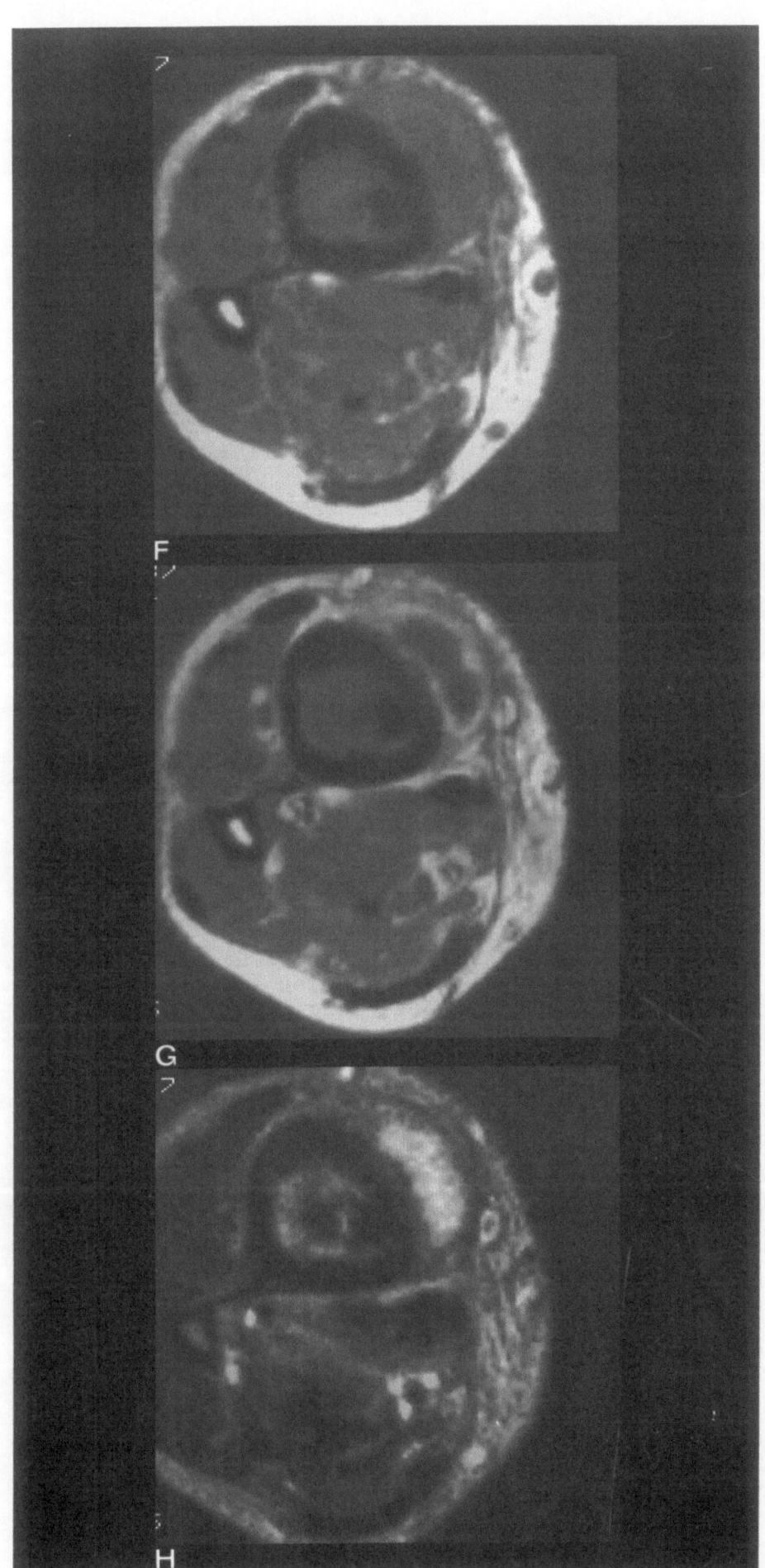

15.3.f, g and h.
MRI, transverse sections at the level of the antero-medial parosteal soft tissue extension.
f. T1-WI
Low SI [3] of the medullary extent, dirty aspect of the permeated cortex. Soft tissue extension appears relatively homogeneous with SI of muscle.
g. T1-WI after intravenous injection of Gd-DTPA.
Definite ringlike enhancement at the periphery of the soft tissue mass. No enhancement at the centre, probably due to intratumoral necrosis.
h. T2-WI.
The tumor extension has an increased SI [7] which is extremely pronounced in the central necrotic region.
Diagnosis: High grade chondrosarcoma.

BENIGN SOFT TISSUE TUMORS

CHAPTER 16

LIPOMA

Lipomas are the most frequently encountered soft tissue tumors, containing fat or fatty components. They are easily recognized on CT by their homogeneous aspect and low attenuation values (-65 to -110 HU). They lack contrast enhancement.
On MRI lipomatous tissue has a high SI [6] on all SE-sequences equal to subcutaneous fat.

COMMENT

We included only two cases of lipoma in our study for illustrative purposes. Histological characterization in both cases was easy as well on CT as on MRI.

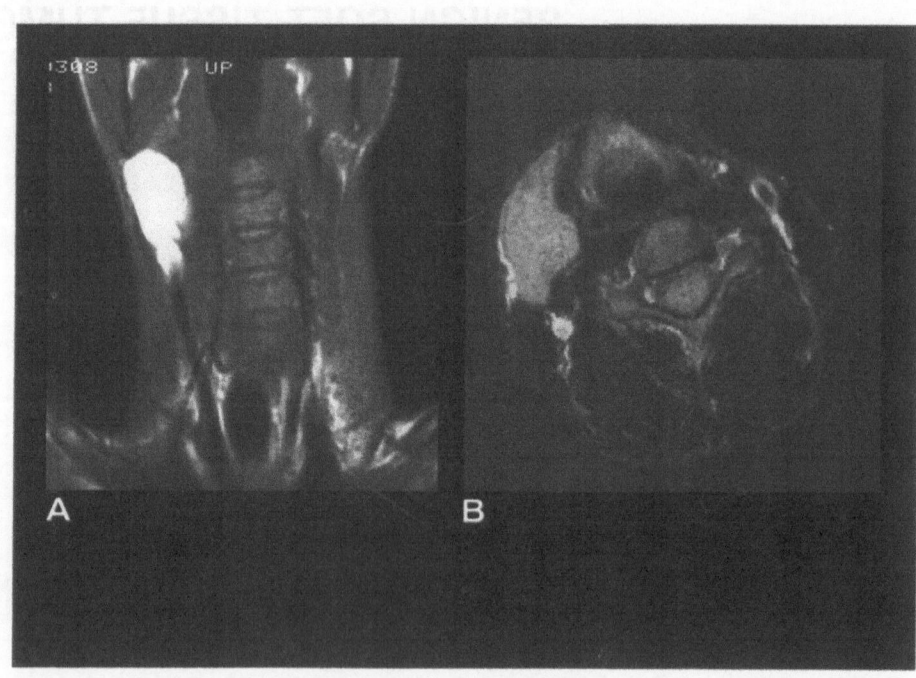

Fig. 16.1. D.L.W., 26 year-old male.

16.1.a. MRI of the neck, coronal section, T1-WI.
Large, well defined mass lesion in the right anterior neck triangle, isointense to subcutaneous fat.
16.1.b. MRI of the neck, transverse section, T2-WI.
The lesion again has the signal intensity of fat [6].
Diagnosis: Lipoma.

NEUROGENIC TUMOR

Tumors of nerves may be solitary or multiple. They may occur in the peripheral, intraspinal or intracranial segment of the nerves.
Histologically they represent proliferation of fibroblasts (neurofibroma) or neurilemmal sheath cells (Schwannoma).
Distinction is made between hypercellular (Anthony A.) and hypocellular tumors (Anthony B.). Both have their own appearance on CT and MRI.
On CT hypocellular or cystic degenerated lesions are rather hypodense. Hypercellular lesions are rather isodense and present with a mottled enhancement pattern after contrast injection (3).
These phenomena are also responsible for MRI findings. When cystic or pseudocystic, they have a low SI on T1- and a high SI on T2-WI. Solid, high cellular lesions as in Schwannoma have an intermediate SI on T1- (>[2] and <[6]) and high SI on T2-WI (>[3] and <[7]) (2).
As reported by Sundaram, the more collagenous, hypocellular lesions presented with a low SI on T2-WI (4).

References

1. Dooms GC, Hricak H, Sollitto RA, Higgins CB. Lipomatous tumors and tumors with fatty component: MR imaging potential and comparison of MR and CT results. Radiology 1985; 157: 479-483.
2. Petasnick JP, Turner DA, Charters JR, Gitelis S, Zacharias CE. Soft-tissue masses of the locomotor system: comparison of MR imaging with CT. Radiology 1986; 160: 125-133.
3. Silver AJ, Mawad ME, Hilal SK, Ascherl GF, Chynn KY, Baredes S. Computed tomography of the carotid space and related cervical spaces. Neurogenic tumors.Radiology 1984; 150: 729-735.
4. Sundaram M, McGuire MH, Schajowicz. Soft-tissue masses: histologic basis for decreased signal (short T2) on T2-weighted MR images. AJR 1987; 148: 1247-1250.

COMMENT

1. Two cases of neurofibromatosis and one case of a Schwannoma are included in our series.

2. Localization and tumor shape (dumbbell) were relatively specific in the case of Schwannoma.

3. In the case of cystic neurofibroma high water content influenced the SI.

4. In the second case of neurofibromatosis (Fig. 16.4) and in the case of Schwannoma (Fig. 16.2) SI was intermediate on T1-[4] and extremely high [8] on T2-WI, reflecting their high cellularity.

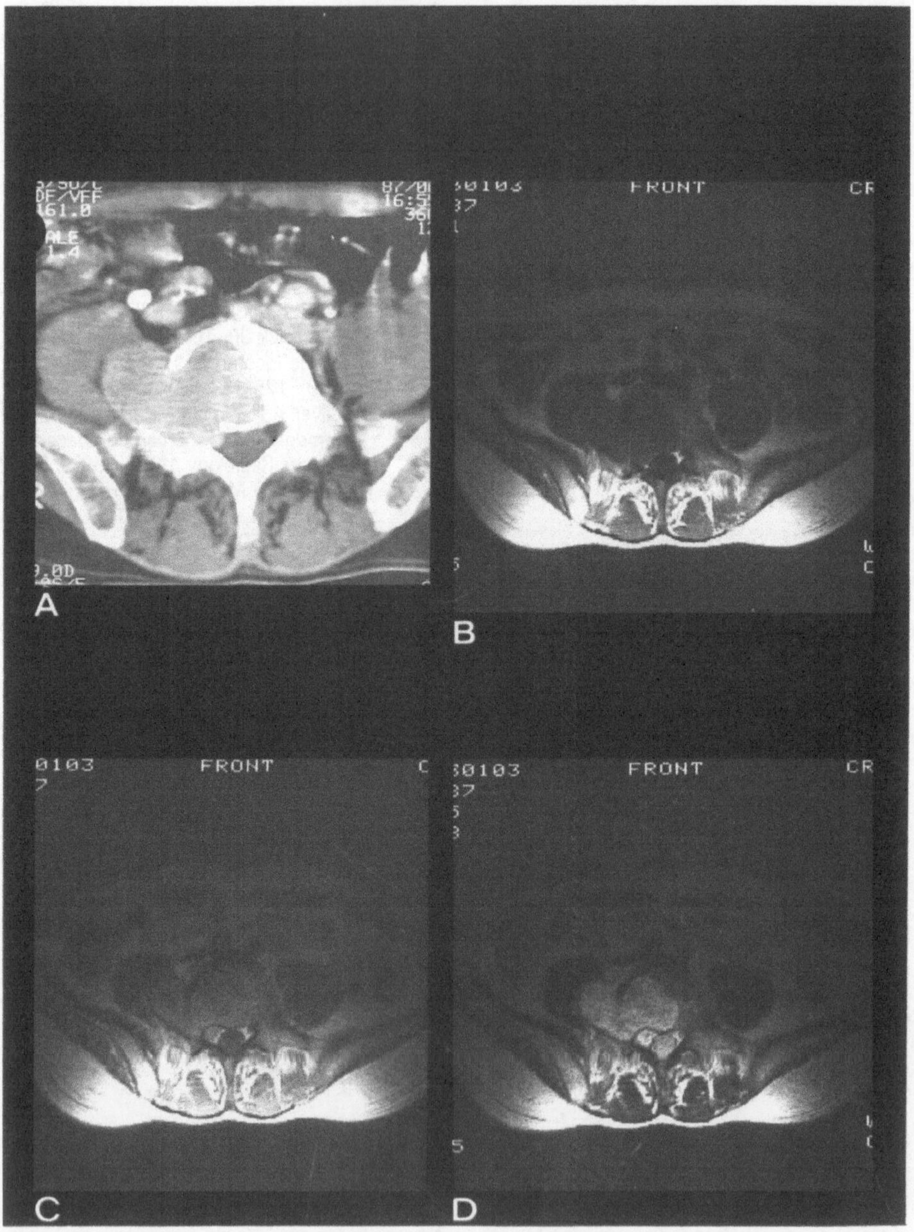

Fig. 16.2. V.H., 54 year-old male.

16.2.a. CT of the lumbar spine, soft tissue
    window.
    Dumbbell-shaped lesion with
    intravertebral and paravertebral
    component eroding the vertebral body
    of LV and extending towards the
    spinal canal with minimal displacement
    of the dural sac. The right psoas
    muscle is displaced by the paravertebral
    extent.
    The lesion is relatively homogeneous
    and hyperdense compared to muscle.
16.2.b. MRI of the lumbar spine, transverse
    section, T1-WI.
    MRI confirms the morphological
    information given by CT. SI is relatively
    uniform and high [4].
16.2.c and d. MRI of the lumbar spine,
    transverse section, proton density-(c)
    and T2-WI (d).
    SI is high on both sequences (up to
    [7] on T2-WI).
Diagnosis: Tumor of the nerve root,
    hypercellular type: Schwannoma.

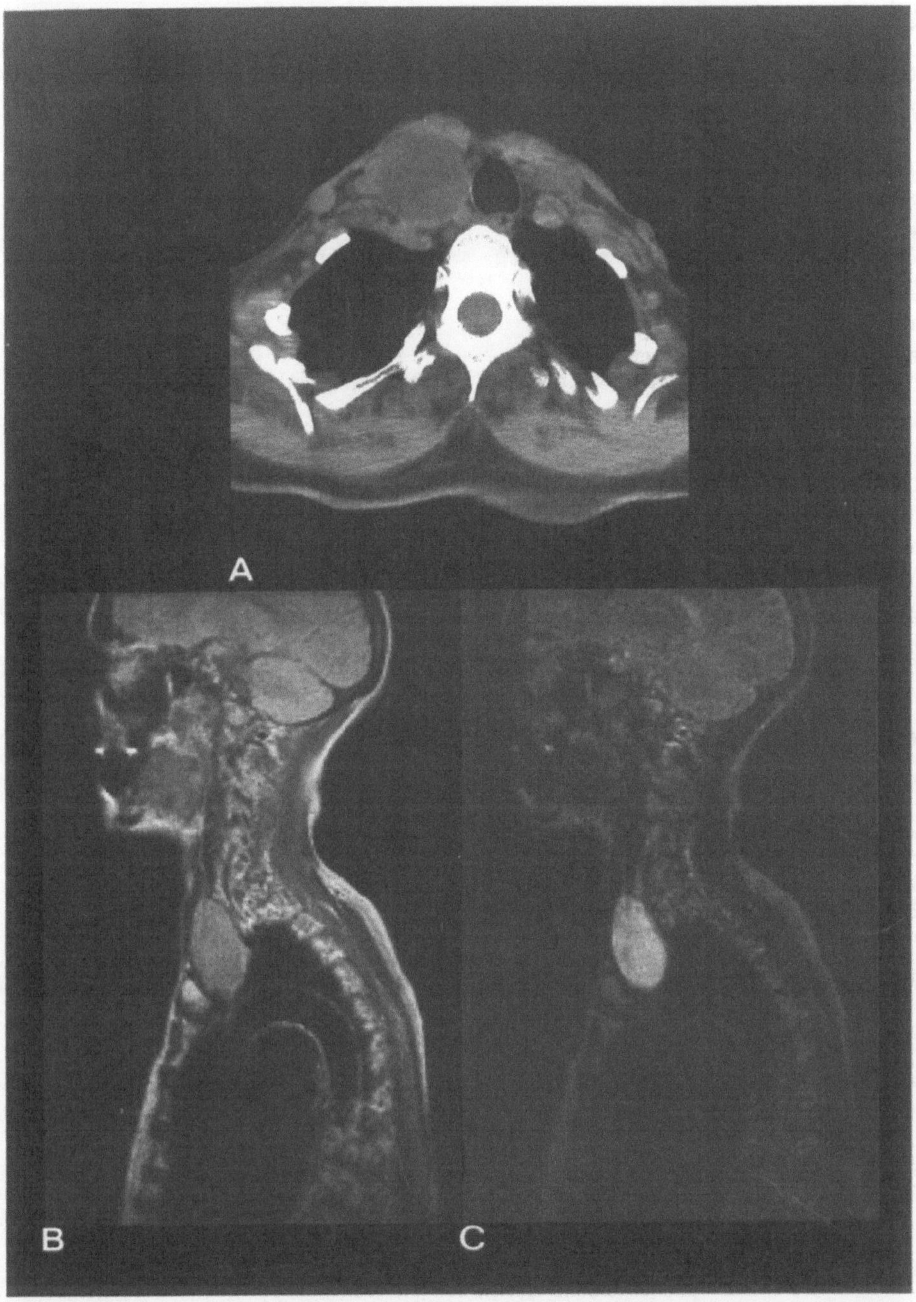

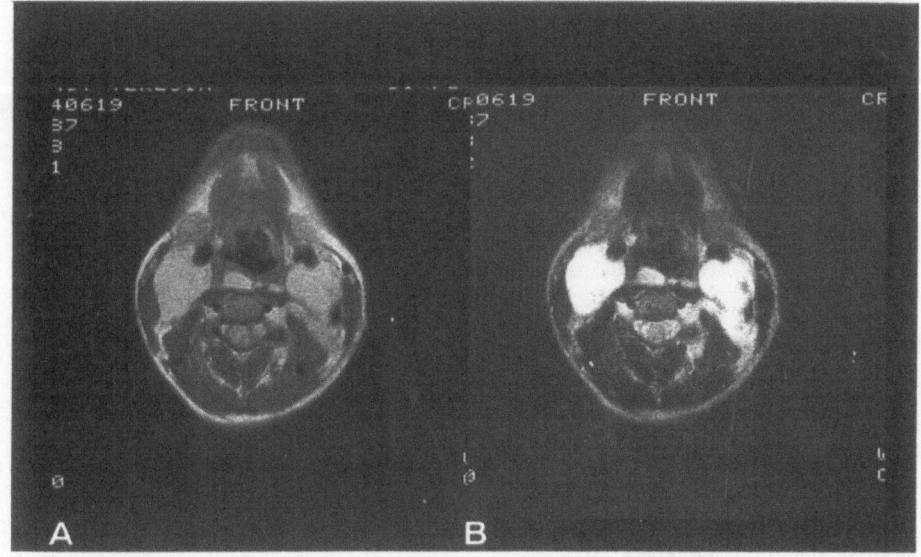

Fig. 16.3. D.M., 66 year-old female.

16.3.a. CT of the lower neck, soft tissue
window.
Rounded, well delineated, mainly
hypodense mass lateral to the trachea
at the level of the thoracic inlet.
16.3.b and c. MRI, sagittal section, proton
density-(b) and T2-WI (c).
Ovoid , well delineated mass with a
very high SI, up to [8] on T2-WI.
Diagnosis: Pseudocystic neurofibroma in
a patient with known neurofibromatosis
and intracranial meningeoma.

Fig. 16.4. V.A.T., 23 year-old female.

16.4.a and b. MRI of the neck, transverse
section, proton density- (a) and T2-WI
(b).
Large tumoral lesions in both carotid
spaces.
SI is homogeneous and extremely
high, up to [8] on T2-WI (intermediate
SI on T1-WI not illustrated).
Diagnosis: Neurofibromas in both carotid
spaces, hypercellular type (Anthony
A.) in a patient with known
neurofibromatosis.

SOFT TISSUE HEMANGIOMA

Soft tissue hemangiomas are uncommon tumors of young adults.
They are characterized by an increased number of vascular channels and
overgrowth of the endothelial lining cells.
In addition to vascular elements adipose, fibrous, muscular and rarely
osseous components are found.
Hemangiomas may be asymptomatic. Rarely they may produce devastating
deformities or lethal complications.
CR, RNSC and CT may not always be specific for this tumor.
CT limited to the axial plane underestimates the extent of the lesion.
Angiography remains a valuable procedure in detection and characterization
of soft tissue hemangiomas and allows a preoperative embolization.
On MRI, hemangiomas have a relatively low, intermediate or high SI on
T1-WI (1) (2). This variable appearance is dependent on their arterial,
capillary or venous nature (different flow characteristics), the presence of
thrombosis, occluded vessels, pooling of large amounts of blood within
the dilated sinuses and various amounts of adipose tissue.
Inhomogeneous pattern of high SI on T2-WI is a constant finding.
Sometimes they present with a serpiginous pattern and focal muscle
atrophy (2).
Margins may be sharp or indistinct, fat or muscle infiltration may or may
not be present.
No contrast studies are reported in the literature.

References

1. Kaplan PA, Williams SM. Mucocutaneous and peripheral soft tissue hemangiomas:
   MR imaging. Radiology 1987; 163: 163-167.
2. Yuh WTC, Kathol MH, Sein MA, Ehara S, Chiu L. Hemangiomas of skeletal
   muscle: MR findings in five patients. AJR 1987; 149: 765-768.

COMMENT

1. One case of soft tissue hemangioma was studied with MRI.

2. MR-findings were in accord with literature data. The lesion was seen
as an intramuscular mass without demonstrable capsule, with a large,
centrally located feeding vessel and of intermediate SI on T1-WI versus
high SI on T2-WI.
No serpiginous pattern or focal muscle atrophy was present in our case.

3. Angiography allowed preoperative embolization aiding the surgeon.

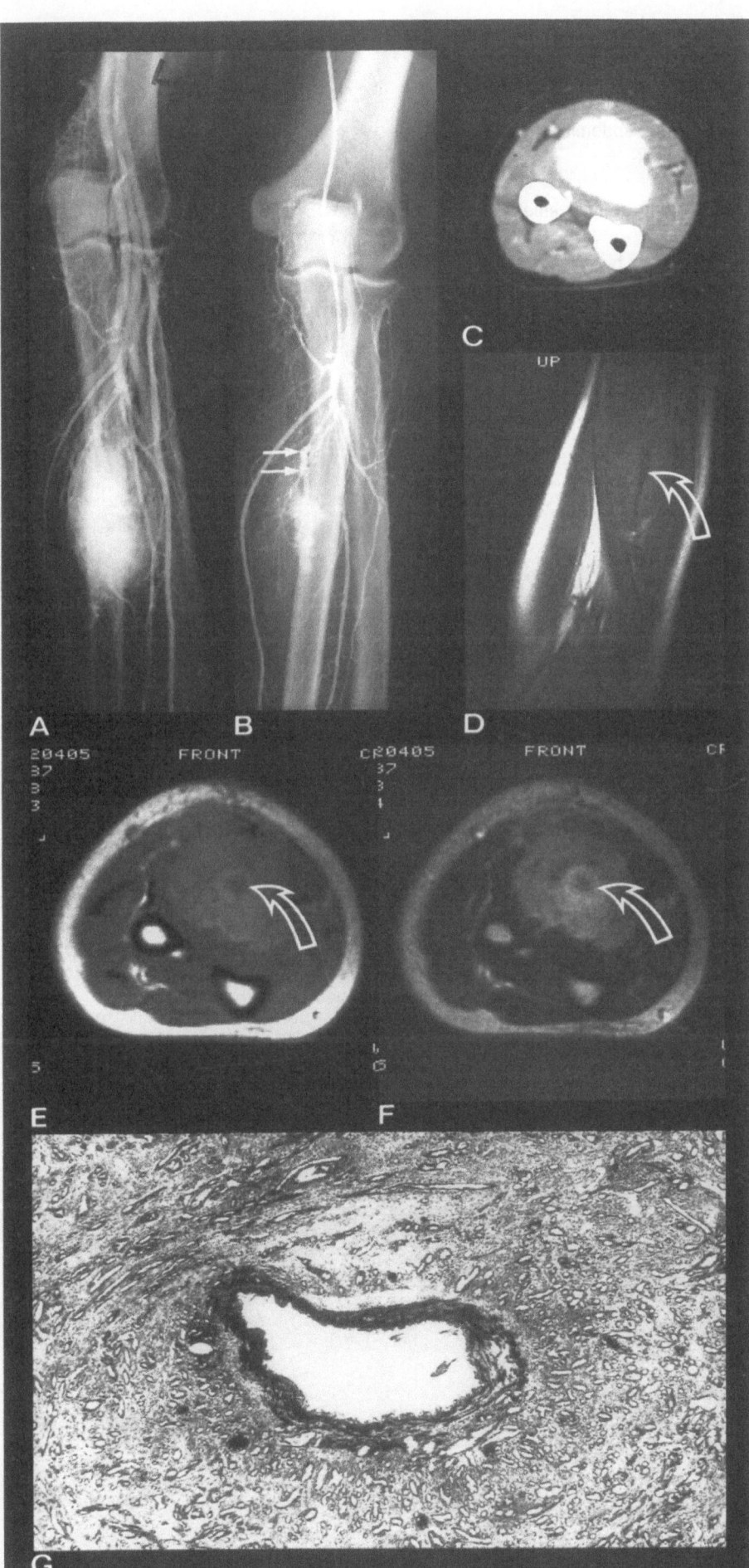

Fig. 16.5. K.M., 55 year-old female.

16.5.a. Angiography of the right brachial
artery.
Highly vascularized mass in the middle
third of the right forearm exclusively
supplied by the enlarged anterior
interosseous artery. There is a
precocious venous drainage.

16.5.b. Control-angiography after
preoperative embolization of the
interosseous artery by means of two
small "Gianturco coils" (arrows).
The procedure accounted for a 90%
devascularization of the tumor facilitating
surgical resection.

16.5.c. CT after injection of contrast
medium.
Hyperdense mass located anteriorly
in the right forearm (flexor muscle).
The lesion margins are well defined,
there is no visible capsule.
Rounded area of lower density in the
centre of the tumor. Radial and ulnar
artery are displaced but not invaded.

16.5.d. MRI, coronal section, T1-WI,
before arterial embolization.
Ovoid, ill defined mass of intermediate
to high SI [4] [5]. Centrally in the
lesion there is a linear structure of
low SI, representing a large intratumoral
vessel (curved open arrow).

16.5.e and f. MRI, transverse section,
proton density-(e) and T2-WI (f).
The lesion remains of high SI [6] with
a central area of low SI (vessel) (curved
open arrow) and no demonstrable
capsule. Highest SI is noted around
the enlarged central vessel.
Inhomogeneity of the subcutaneous
fat on the anterior part of the forearm
is due to a previous biopsy.

16.5.g. Microphotograph.
Tumoral tissue contains a large number
of vascular channels forming a capillary
hemangioma. Large central vessel.

Diagnosis: Intramuscular hemangioma
with enlarged central vessel with high
blood flow.

AGGRESSIVE FIBROMATOSIS

Aggressive fibromatosis is a tumorlike condition occurring mostly in young adults. The lesion has the histology of a fibroma (benign proliferation of fibrous tissue) but is not encapsulated. It infiltrates the surrounding muscles, destroying the muscle fibres. It often recurs locally after excision but never metastasises. Most frequent localizations are the rectus abdominis muscle, shoulder and thigh region and upper portion of the back.

The tumoral mass may be clinically tender and painful.

CR and RNSC are of little value except for the detection of involvement of adjacent bone.

On CT, without contrast injection, the lesions are slightly hypodense or isodense with respect to the muscle. After contrast injection they show an intense enhancement.

On MRI aggressive fibromatosis is described as a low SI-lesion on both SE-sequences (1) (5).

Conversely, Bloem reported 4 cases presenting a high SI on T2-WI (2). According to Sundaram this is caused by high cellularity and an increased amount of intracellular water (4).

COMMENT

1. One case of aggressive fibromatosis (two locations) is included in our series.

2. The lesions exhibited the CT-characteristics as mentioned before.

3. The primary lesion in the gluteal region had the SI's described in the literature and shows a moderate enhancement after Gd-DTPA-injection.

4. The recurrent lesion in the thigh presented with a peripheral fibrous component (low SI on both SE-sequences) and a central more cellular component with the same SI's as the primary gluteal lesion as well before as after contrast injection.

The same two components with identical SI's were seen in a case reported by Petasnick (3).

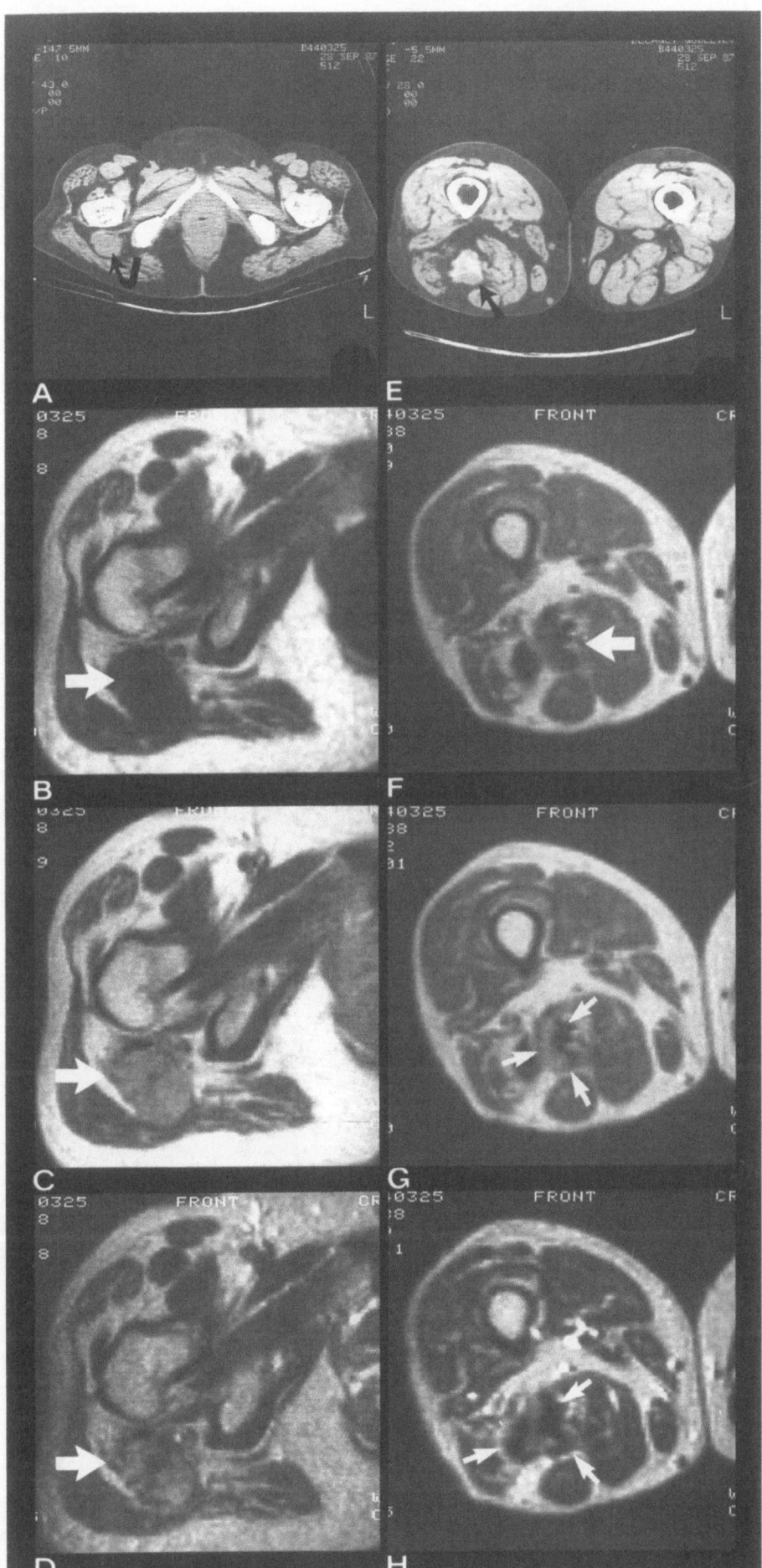

Fig. 16.6. D.G., 43 year-old female.

16.6.a. CT at the level of the ischial
tuberosity, soft tissue window.
Rounded, well delineated mass between
trochanteric bone, gluteus maximus
muscle and ischial tuberosity (curved
arrow).
The mass is homogeneous and has
a muscle density.

16.6.b, c and d. MRI of the gluteal region,
transverse section (same level as CT-
Fig. 16.6.a.)
b. T1-WI.
Lobulated well delineated mass with
SI of muscle [3] (arrow). The lesion
is clearly separated from the sciatic
nerve.
c. T1-WI, after intravenous injection
of Gd-DTPA.
Enhancement is responsible for increase
in SI up to [5] (arrow).
d. T2-WI.
Inhomogeneous aspect of the lesion
with an intermediate SI [4] (arrow).

16.6.e. CT at the level of the middle third
of the thigh, after contrast injection,
soft tissue window.
Rounded mass with slightly irregular
margins located between the biceps
femoris muscle, adductor muscles
and hamstrings (arrow). There is a
moderate enhancement of the central
portion of the lesion.

16.6.f, g and h. MRI of the thigh region,
transverse section (same level as CT-
Fig. 16.6.e).
f. T1-WI.
Triangular mass with a low SI of the
periphery and an intermediate SI of
the central area [3] (arrow).
g. T1-WI after injection of Gd-DTPA.
Slight enhancement of the central
portion of the lesion up to SI [5].
No enhancement of the peripheral rim.
h. T2-WI.
The peripheral part of the lesion
generates no signal while the central
area is of intermediate SI [4] [5] (arrow).

Diagnosis: Aggressive fibromatosis with
a recurrent lesion in the thigh and a
new lesion in the gluteal region.
Both lesions illustrate different aspects
of aggressive fibromatosis.

MALIGNANT SOFT TISSUE TUMORS

CHAPTER 17

LIPOSARCOMA

Liposarcoma is the most frequently encountered soft tissue tumor in adults. The mean age of the patients is about 50 years. Men are more often affected than women. Tumors are preferentially located in the gluteal, femoral and retroperitoneal area.

Histologically liposarcomas are classified as grade I: well differentiated liposarcomas or lipoma-like sarcomas; grade II: myxoid liposarcomas, grade III: "round cell" liposarcomas and grade IV: pleiomorphic liposarcomas.

Mitotic activity increases, cell differentiation decreases and metastatic potential increases with tumor grade.

Unlike lipomas, liposarcomas mostly present on CR-CT as voluminous masses with inconstant density depending on their histological nature.

On MRI, grade I-tumors have SI's comparable to subcutaneous fat on both SE-sequences. SI on T1-WI decreases and SI on T2-WI increases with malignancy grade.

There is also an increase in tumor heterogeneity with increase of the malignancy grade. As a consequence, MRI has a potential value not only in detecting and staging but also in predicting histological grading.

Liposarcomas have a lobular structure. Lobules are separated by septa having low SI on both SE-sequences, indicating their fibrous character. Postoperative fibrotic scar tissue has a low SI as well on T1- as on T2-WI, allowing differentiation with postoperative tumor recurrence.

No contrast studies are published in current literature.

References

1. Bloem JL.Radiological staging of primary musculoskeletal tumors. Proefschrift, 's Gravenhage, 1988.
2. Dooms GC, Hricak H, Sollitto RA, Higgins CB. Lipomatous tumors and tumors with fatty component: MR imaging potential and comparison of MR and CT results. Radiology 1985; 157: 479-483.
3. Moon KL, Genant HK, Helms CA, Chafetz NI, Crooks LE, Kaufman L. Musculosketal applications of nuclear magnetic resonance. Radiology 1983; 147: 161-171.
4. Petterson H, Springfield DS, Enneking WF. Radiological management of musculoskeletal tumors. Springer-Verlag. London Berlin Heidelberg New York Paris Tokio, 1987.
5. Richardson ML, Kilcoyne RF, Gillespy III T, Helms CA, Genant HK. Magnetic resonance imaging of musculoskeletal neoplasms. Radiol Clin North Am 1986; 24(2): 259-267.

COMMENT

1. Four cases of liposarcoma are included in our study. They were illustrative for the different histological grades of this tumor.

2. Three tumors were located in the femoral region and one in the popliteal fossa. Two tumors had an intramuscular and two others had an intermuscular localization.

3. All lesions were lobulated, interspersed by fibrous septa and sharply demarcated.

4. Relationship with adjacent bone, neurovascular structures and muscles was well illustrated. Microscopic osseous involvement (reactive) in case Fig. 17.1. could not be demonstrated on MRI (grade I liposarcoma II)

110

5.SI on T1-WI decreased and SI on T2-WI increased with increasing of myxoid and/or sarcomatous nature of the lobules. Fat lobules were of high SI on T1-WI and intermediate SI on T2-WI.
As a consequence fat lobules were easily differentiated by SI from myxoid, sarcomatous and fibrous nodules in all cases.
In this regard MRI not only has a potential value in detecting and staging but also in predicting histological grading of liposarcomas.

6. Extensive enhancement of myxoid and sarcomatous nodules after contrast injection seemed related to SI-increase on T2-WI.
MR-grey scale of Liposarcoma, see chapter 19.

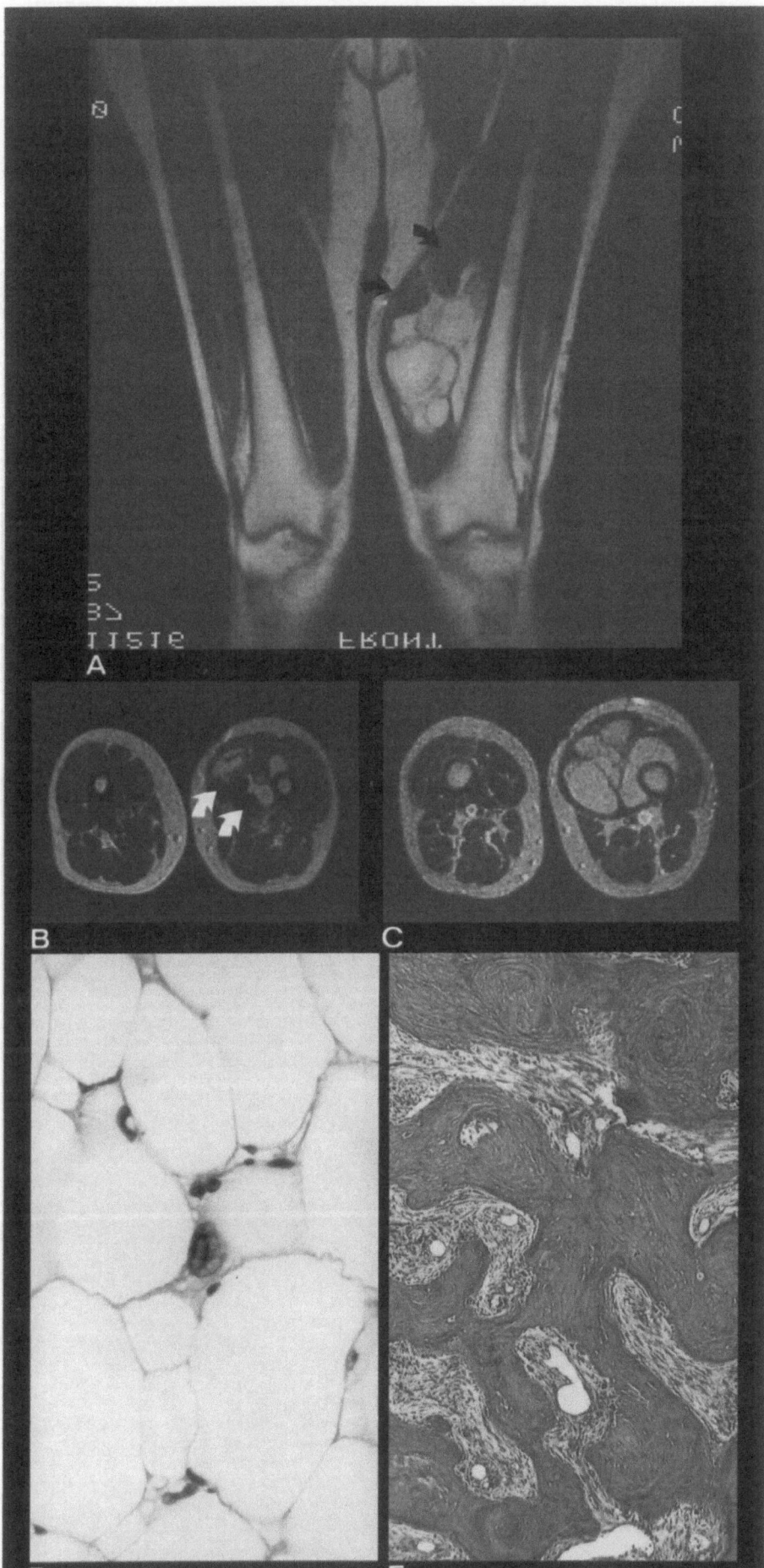

Fig. 17.1. M.L., 66 year-old female.

17.1.a. MRI of the left thigh, coronal
    section T1-WI.
    Multilobulated mass in the left vastus
    medialis muscle with a diameter of
    10 x 7 cm. Most lobules are isointense
    with respect to subcutaneous fat. In
    the cranial part of the lesion some
    nodules generate no visible signal
    (curved arrows). The lesion does not
    disrupt the muscular fascia. Adjacent
    cortical bone has a normal, extremely
    low SI.
17.1.b. MRI of the thigh, transverse
    section, proton density image.
    Section at the level of the cranial part
    of the mass.
    Again lobules with high SI and lobules
    without signal are demonstrated
    (curved arrows).
17.1.c. MRI of the thigh, transverse
    section, T2-WI.
    Section at the level of the caudal part
    of the mass.
    All tumoral lobules have the same
    high SI on this section.
17.1.d and e. Microphotographs (Courtesy
    Dr.Bultinck, Antwerp).
    d. High power microphotograph.
    In the centre abnormal lipocyte with
    a large nucleus and nucleolus. The
    other lipocytes are of unequal size.
    e. Low power microphotograph.
    Reactive hyperplasia and fibrosis of
    the marrow cavities in the adjacent
    bone.
Diagnosis: Recurrent liposarcoma (grade
    I). Lobules without signal on both
    SE-sequences are thought to be of
    fibrous nature.

112

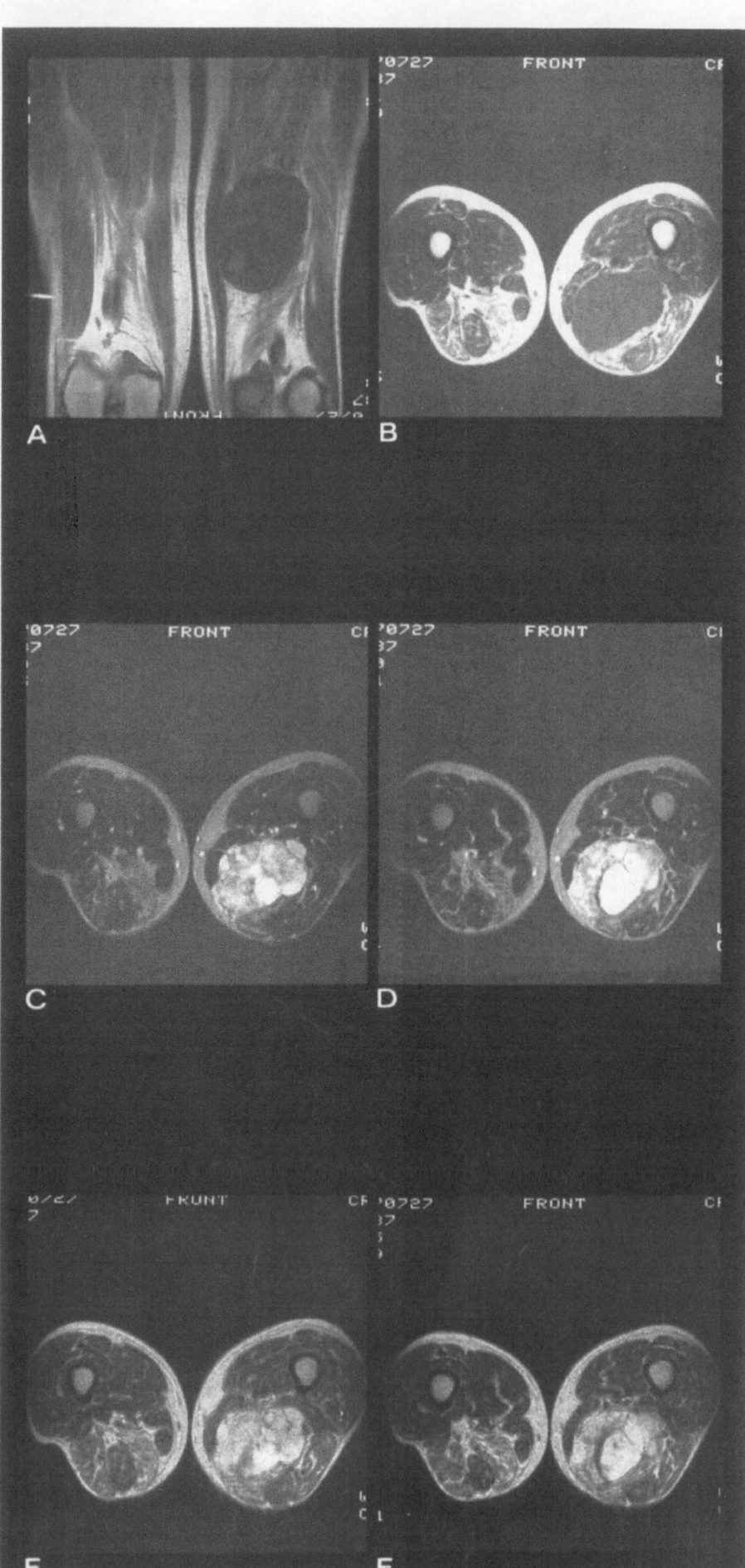

Fig. 17.2. E.E., 51 year-old female.

17.2.a. MRI of the thigh, coronal section,
T1-WI.
Large, rounded multilobulated and
sharply delineated mass in the left
femoral region. The tumor is located
between the gracilis and sartorius
muscle on one side and the hamstrings
on the other side. Tumor lobules are
of different SI but mean SI is low [1] [2].

17.2.b. MRI of the thigh, transverse
section, T1-WI.
The relationship with adjacent
neurovascular elements and adjacent
muscle groups is easy to evaluate on
this section.

17.2.c and d. MRI of the thigh, transverse
section, T2-WI.
Multilobulated aspect is well
demonstrated on this series. Tumoral
lobules are of high SI [7] [8] while
interspersed septa generate no signal.

17.2.e and f. MRI of the thigh, transverse
section, T1-WI after intravenous
injection of Gd-DTPA .
There is an intense enhancement of
the tumoral nodules.

Diagnosis: Myxoid liposarcoma (grade II).

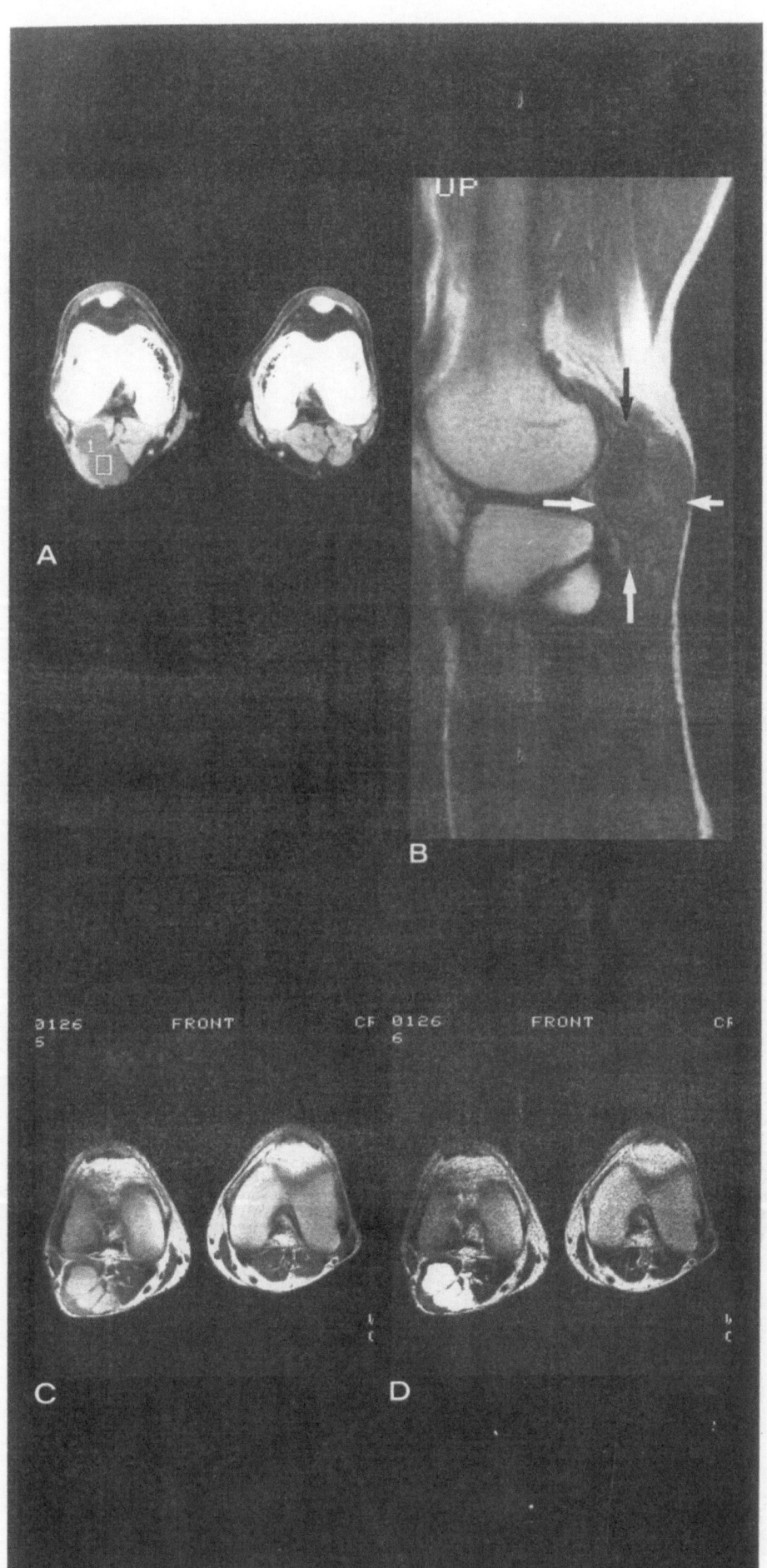

Fig. 17.3. V.O.L., 42 year-old male.

17.3.a. CT at knee level (soft tissue
    window).
    Bilobulated, sharply delineated,
    homogeneous mass located in the
    lateral head of the right gastrocnemic
    muscle. The lesion has a mean density
    of 23 H.U..
17.3.b. MRI at knee level, sagittal section,
    T1-WI.
    Multilobulated mass in the right popliteal
    fossa (arrows). SI of the tumor is
    comparable to SI of adjacent normal
    muscle [2][3], and consequently the
    tumoral margins are less conspicuous.
    Tumor lobules have a variable SI.
17.3.c and d. MRI at knee level, transverse
    section, proton density-(c) and T2-WI
    (d).
    Tumor lobules are of high SI on T2-WI
    and separated by low SI septa.
    Due to the decreased SI of adjacent
    muscle on T2-WI the limits of the
    tumoral mass are clearly outlined.
    Relationship with adjacent vascular
    structures and knee joint are well
    demonstrated.
Diagnosis: Myxoid-round cell liposarcoma
    (Type II-III).

114

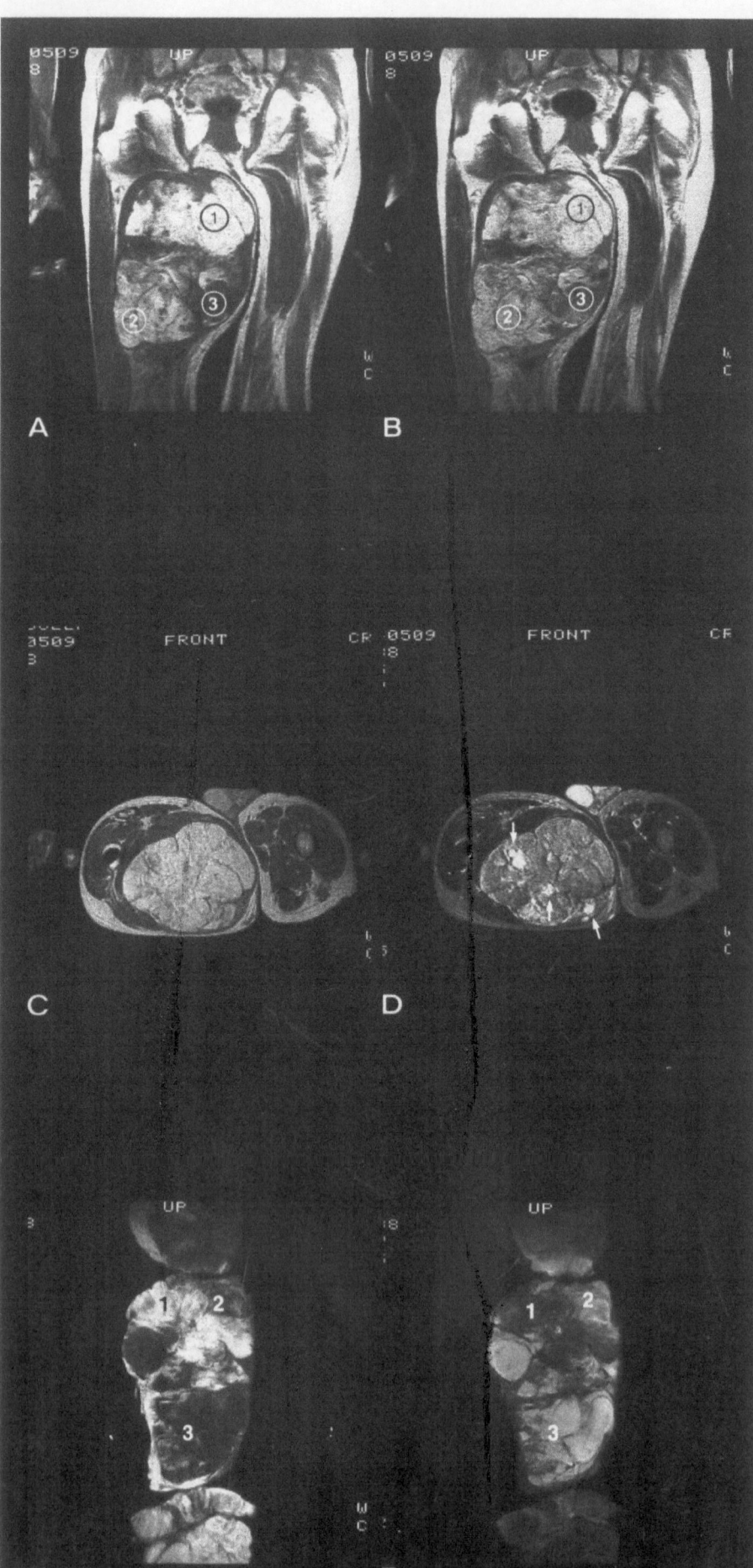

Fig. 17.4. D.V.J., 68 year-old male.

17.4.a. MRI of the thigh, coronal section,
T1-WI.
Large, polylobulated soft tissue mass
in the right thigh. Tumor lobules have
a variable SI from extremely high [8]
(area 1) over intermediate [4] (area
2) to very low [2] (area 3).

17.4.b. MRI of the thigh, coronal section,
T1-WI after intravenous injection of
Gd-DTPA.
No visible enhancement in area 1,
intermediate more uniform enhancement
in area 2 and ringlike enhancement
in area 3.

17.4.c and d. MRI of the thigh, transverse
section, proton density-(c) and T2-WI
(d), section at the level of area 1.
Uniform, high SI on proton density
image and less uniform high SI on
T2-WI. Small areas of higher SI [8]
represent myxoid tissue (arrowheads).
Tumoral mass is sharply demarcated
with normal appearance of the adjacent
muscles.

17.4.e and f. MRI of the operative specimen.
Illustration of different tumor
components with corresponding SI
on T1-(e) and T2-WI (f).

Diagnosis: Liposarcoma with lipomatous
(area 1), myxoid (area 2) and
pleiomorphic (area 3) components.
(see also chapter 1, Fig. 1.4.)

CHAPTER 18

MALIGNANT FIBROUS HISTIOCYTOMA

Together with pleiomorphic liposarcomas and pleiomorphic rhabdomyosarcomas malignant fibrous histiocytomas are the most frequently encountered malignant soft tissue tumors.

Mean age of the patients is about 60 years. There is no sex relation. They are preferentially located in the thigh and the extremities, deeply within muscle or superficially within subcutaneous fat.

Biological behaviour depends on anatomic site and location.

Recurrence is seen in 37-51% after complete excision. Overall 5-year survival rate is 36%. Histologically they have a pleiomorphic appearance with spindle cells, oval and round cells, benign and malignant giant cells. They are subclassified as fibrous (65%), giant cell, myxoid or inflammatory variants (1, 2).

Destruction of adjacent bone structures is present in 20% of the cases, while peripheral calcifications are seen in 9%.

Both features are easily demonstrated on CR-CT. On CT the lesion has an intermediate density (40-60 H_xU_x), is inhomogeneous and ill defined.

On MRI the lesion presents with characteristic signs of malignancy i.e. indistinct margins, non uniform SI which is relatively high on both T1-and T2-images. Low SI on T2-WI is reported by Sundaram and thought to be caused by low cellularity and high content of collagen (4).

Peritumoral edema, joint effusion or invasion and intratumoral necrosis are well demonstrated (3, 5).

References

1. Antoni F , Capanna R, Biagini R et al.Malignant fibrous histiocytoma of soft tissue.Cancer 1985; 56: 356-367.
2. Kearny MM, Soule EH, Ivins JC.Malignant fibrous histiocytoma. Cancer 1980; 45: 167-178.
3. Pettersson H, Gillespy III T, Hamlin DJ, Enneking WF et all. Primary musculoskeletal tumors: examination with MR imaging compared with conventional modalities. Radiology 1987; 164: 237-241.
4. Sundaram M, McGuire MH, Schajowicz. Soft-tissue masses: histologic basis for decreased signal (short T2) on T2-weighted MR images. AJR 1987; 148: 1247-1250.
5. Wetzel LH, Levine E, Murphey MD. A comparison of MR imaging and CT in the evaluation of musculoskeletal masses. RadioGraphics 1987; 7(5): 851-874.

COMMENT

1. Two cases of malignant fibrous histiocytoma were studied with MRI.

2. They both presented themselves on MRI with characteristic morphological signs of malignancy.

3. SI's were in concordance with literature data.
According to Sundaram's statement that the histologic composition of the tumor rather than the histologic diagnosis appears to influence the MR signal on T2-WI, both tumors are expected to be relatively cellular and to contain a small amount of fibrous tissue. This was confirmed by histology. The lower SI on T2-WI of the intrapelvic soft tissue component in case 18.2 is presumed to be caused by rather low cellularity and the presence of more fibrous tissue (4).

4. Minimal enhancement was seen after injection of Gd-DTPA.
MR-grey scale of malignant fibrous histiocytoma, see chapter 19.

116

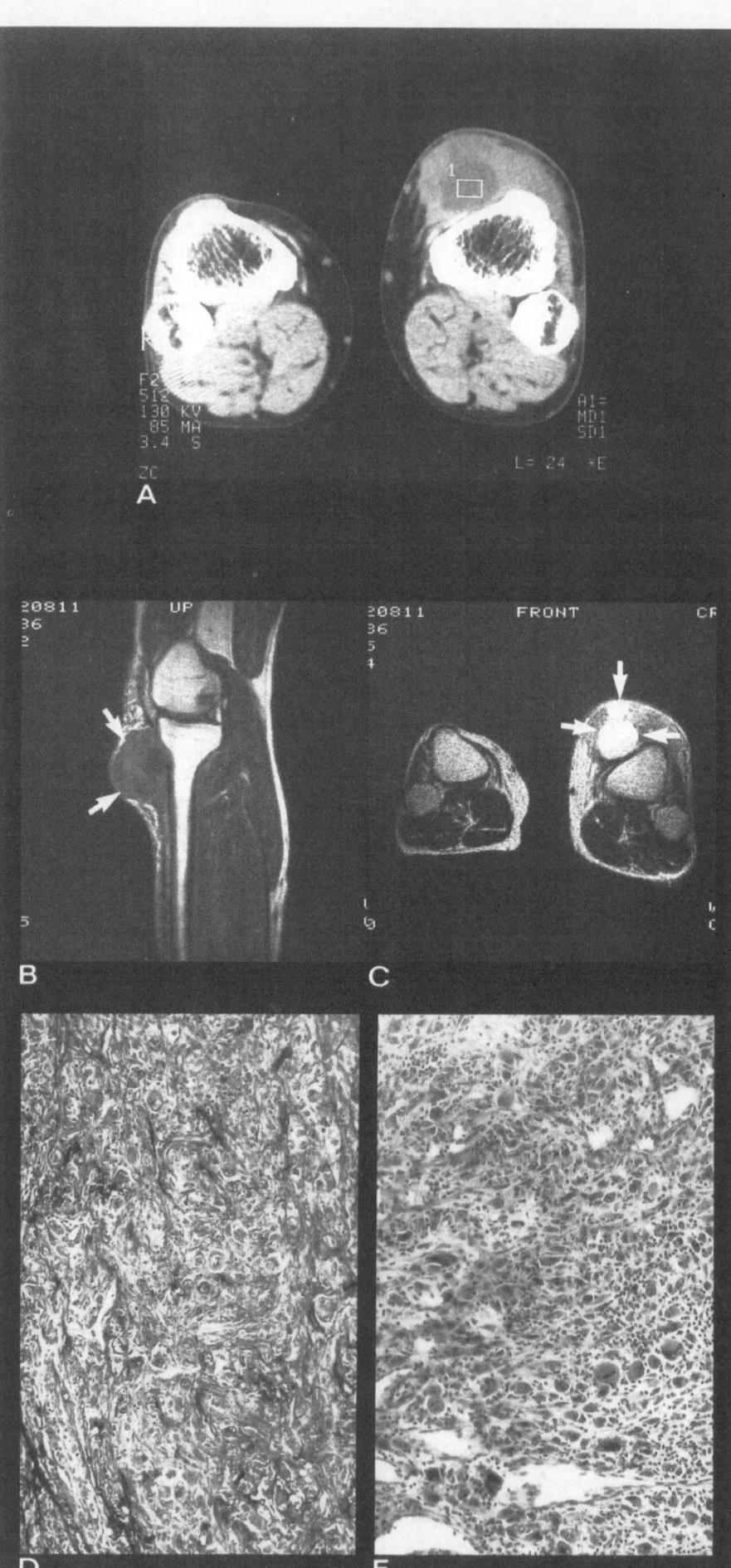

Fig. 18.1. V.H.A., 75 year-old male.

18.1.a. CT at knee level.
  Pretibial mass with a central low-density area, consistent with necrosis and liquefaction. Preserved fat plane between the tumor and the anterior cortex of the tibia.

18.1.b. MRI of the left knee, sagittal section, T1-WI.
  Pretibial mass with ill defined transition between tumor and subcutaneous fat (arrows). Anterior cortex of the tibia seems intact. The overall SI is slightly higher than that of muscle [4] but is non uniform.
  Besides the low SI areas [2] (intratumoral necrosis) there are some foci of higher SI [5].

18.1.c. MRI at knee level, transverse section, T2-WI.
  The soft tissue mass has an intermediate [5] and slightly inhomogeneous SI while central areas of necrosis present with a high SI [8] (arrows). Intact anterior tibial cortex.

18.1.d and e. Microphotograph.
  d. Abnormal fibroblasts, some of which are multinucleated intermingled with bundles of collagen fibers.
  e. Cellular part of the same tumor showing many large multinucleated cells.
Diagnosis: Malignant fibrous histiocytoma.

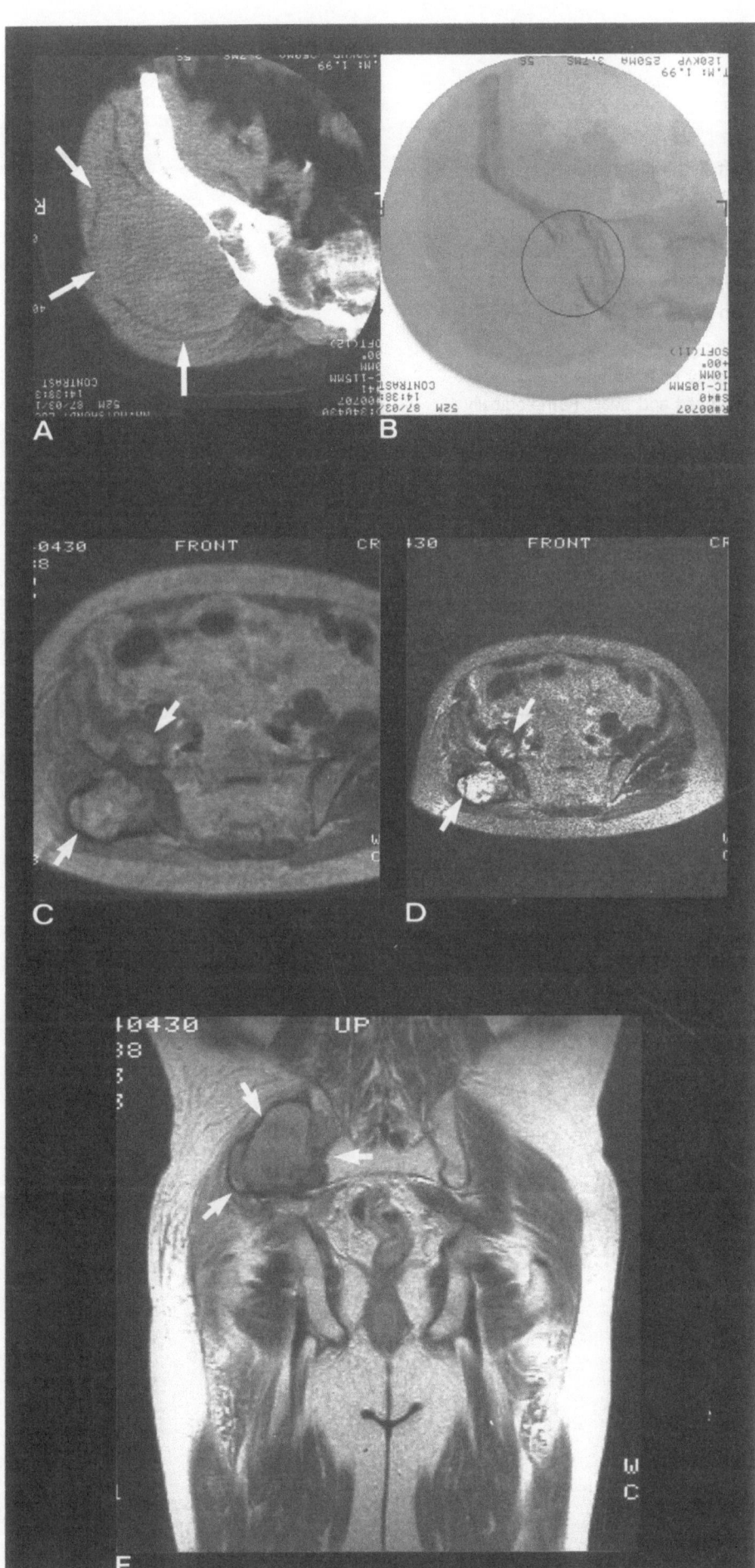

Fig. 18.2. M.L., 64 year-old male.

18.2.a. CT of the right pelvis, soft tissue window.
   Large, well defined soft tissue mass in the right gluteal region (arrows). The tumor is slightly inhomogeneous and has a density comparable with that of muscle.
18.2.b. CT of the right pelvis, bone window. Destruction of adjacent cortical bone (encircled).
18.2.c and d. MRI of the pelvis, transverse section, proton density-(c) and T2-WI (d).
   Presence of tumor extent on both sides of the iliac bone (arrows). On T2-WI the extrapelvic portion is relatively homogeneous and has a high SI [8] while the intrapelvic component has a lower, inhomogeneous SI [3] [4].
   Pathological bone has a low SI [3].
18.2.e. MRI of the pelvis, coronal section, T1-WI after intravenous injection of Gd-DTPA.
   There is no visible enhancement of the soft tissue component and only minimal enhancement of the osseous component of the lesion.
Diagnosis: Malignant fibrous histiocytoma.
   The case illustrates one of the MRI-characteristics of a malignant tumor i.e.
   circumferential growth around osseous structures.

CHAPTER 19

RHABDOMYOSARCOMA

Rhabdomyosarcomas represent 20% of all soft tissue sarcomas.
Histologically and clinically there are three types.

1) The embryonal type is mostly seen in infants and young children. Facial
bones are the preferential localization. The tumor presents itself as a
nodular, well circumscribed or poorly defined mass.
Pathologically long spindle cells are arranged in parallel or interlacing
bundles.

2) The alveolar type is mostly encountered in older children and young
adults, preferentially located at the extremities, head and neck. Pathologically
predominant cells are round and often mixed with multinucleated giant cells.
The alveolar pattern is produced by the tendency of the cells to line
irregularly connective tissue septa.

3) The pleiomorphic type represents 10% of all rhabdomyosarcomas. The
tumor is seen in adults and is mostly localized in the skeletal muscles. It
is the largest of the three types and usually exhibits extensive hæmorrhage
and necrosis.
Spindle shaped cells in parallel or interlacing bundles or without any special
pattern, multinucleated giant cells, strap and racquet shaped cells make
the pleiomorphic pattern of the tumor (1).

Whereas CR, ultrasound and angiography are of little value in detection,
diagnosis and staging of embryonic rhabdomyosarcomas, CT has a
substantial contribution to the diagnosis by showing the soft tissue mass,
the bone destruction especially at the skull base, orbital walls and walls
of the maxillary sinuses. CT also contributes to the follow-up during
treatment. It shows the efficacity of treatment, confirms the diagnosis of
complete remission and is valuable in evaluation of recurrence (2).

Zimmer reports the MR-findings in a case of rhabdomyosarcoma which
has the longest calculated T1-relaxation time in a series of 13 soft tissue
tumors (3). To our knowledge no other cases of rhabdomyosarcomas are
reported.

References

1. Albores-Saavedra J,Martin RG, Smith JL.Rhabdomyosarcoma: study of 35 cases.
   Annals of Surgery 1963; 157: 186-197.
2. Geoffray A, Vanel D, Masselot J et al. Contribution of computed tomography
   in tho otudy of 24 head and neck embryonic rhabdomyosarcomas in children.
   Europ J Radiol 1984; 4: 177-180.
3. Zimmer WD, Berquist TH, McLeod RA, Sim FH et all. Bone tumors: magnetic
   resonance imaging versus computed tomography. Radiology 1985; 155: 709-718.

COMMENT

1. Two cases of rhabdomyosarcoma were studied by MRI. One case of embryonal sarcoma in a young child and another case of pleiomorphic sarcoma in an elderly woman.

2. In the first case CR-CT demonstrated better osseous invasion of the ramus mandibulae while SI of the lesion was aspecific.

3. In the second case pleiomorphism was best demonstrated after contrast injection as well on CT as on MRI.

4. In both cases an extremely high SI on T2-WI [8] was noted.

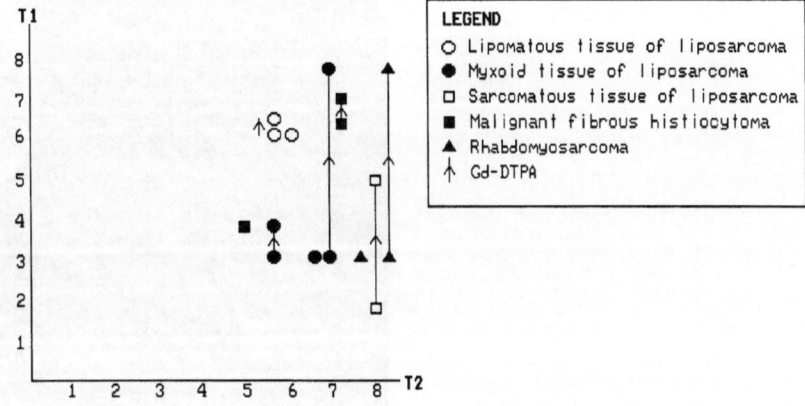

120

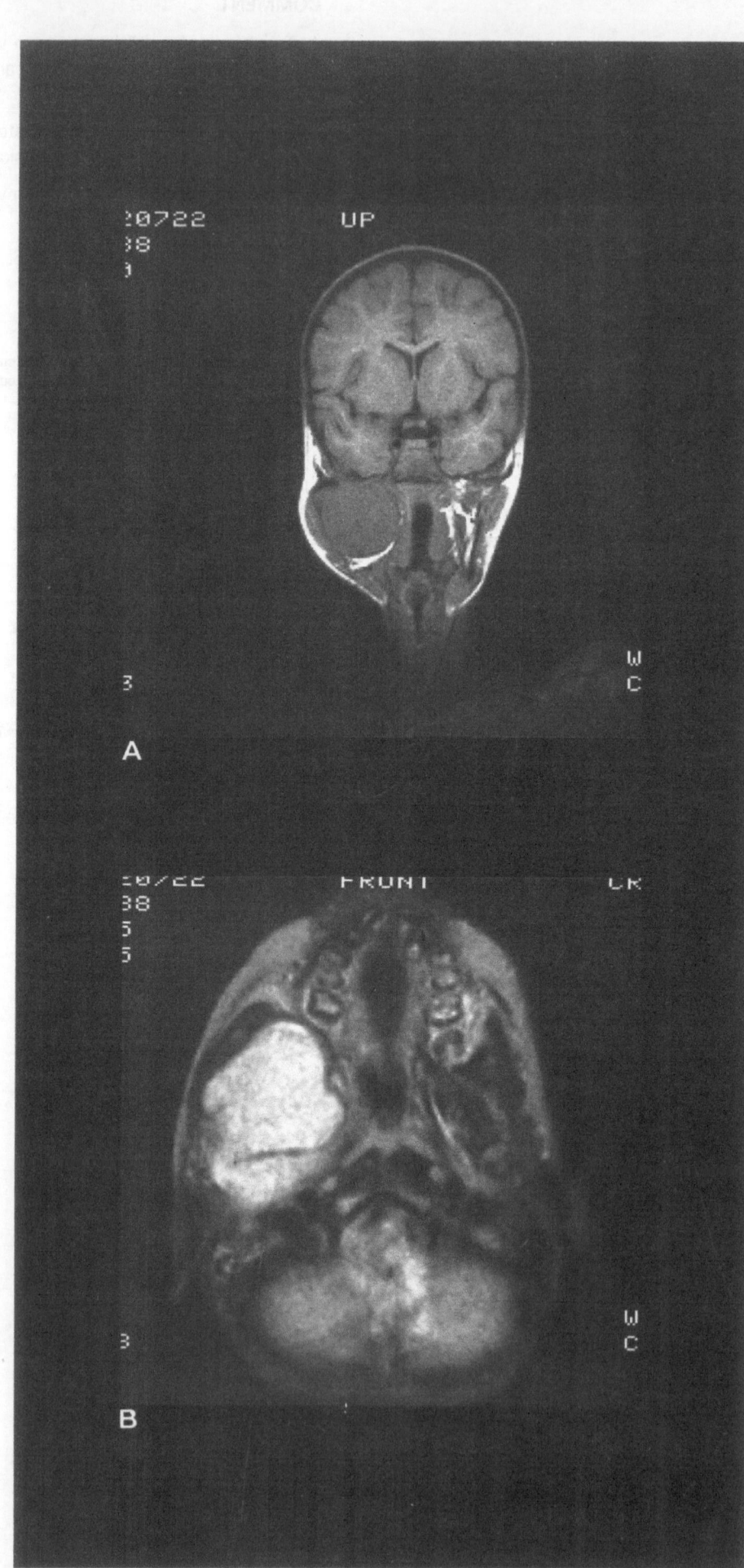

Fig. 19.1. D.K.L., 6 year-old female.

19.1.a. MRI, coronal section, T1-WI.
Large, rounded mass in the region of
the right ramus mandibulae.
The lesion has an intermediate [3],
slightly inhomogeneous SI.
Invasion and destruction of the right
mandibula (better demonstrated on
CR and CT) with loss of differentiation
between cortex and medulla.
19.1.b. MRI, transaxial section, T2-WI.
Extremely high SI of the lesion [8].
Lateral tumor margins are poorly
delineated.
Diagnosis: Embryonal type of
rhabdomyosarcoma.

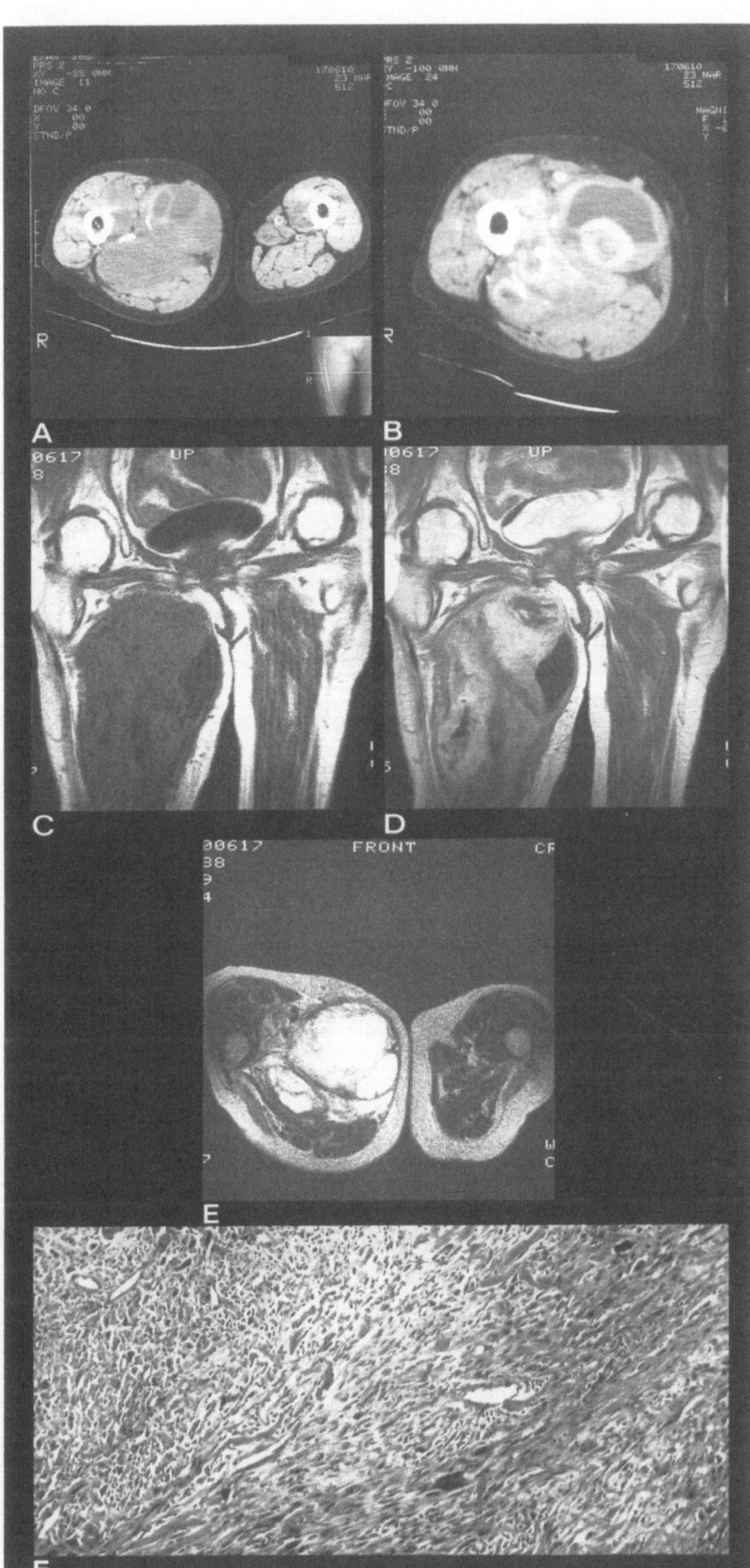

Fig. 19.2. V.M., 78 year-old female.

19.2.a and b. CT of the right thigh at different levels, before (a) and after (b) contrast injection.
Multilobulated, inhomogeneous, mainly hypodense mass invading several thigh muscles (adductor magnus et longus, vastus medialis and biceps femoris muscles).
Intense, mostly ringlike enhancement after contrast injection. Areas of no enhancement are presumably caused by intratumoral necrosis.

19.2.c. MRI of the right thigh, coronal section, T1-WI.
The full extent of the mass is exactly defined on coronal plane. Main SI is comparable with SI of normal muscle [3] but areas of slightly increased and decreased SI are present [2] [4].

19.2.d. MRI of the right thigh, coronal section, T1-WI, after intravenous injection of Gd-DTPA.
At least four different types of enhancement are seen on this sequence. Medially there is a rhomboid area of no enhancement (intratumoral necrosis); cranially there is an area of intensive, homogeneous enhancement; laterally an area of intense ringlike enhancement is seen and caudally there is a ringlike enhancement of lower intensity.

19.2.e. MRI of the thigh region, transverse section, T2-WI.
All tumor components with inclusion of the necrotic areas, have an extremely high SI [8].

19.2.f. Microphotograph (Courtesy Dr. Van Marck, Antwerp).
Strands of abnormal, fusiform cells, some of which contain abundant cytoplasm and large, irregular nuclei.

Diagnosis: Rhabdomyosarcoma, pleiomorphic type.
Morphological signs are indicative of a malignant tumor.
Pleiomorphic nature is best demonstrated after intravenous injection of Gd-DTPA.

CHAPTER 20

VALUE OF CONTRAST
(Gd-DTPA)-ENHANCED MRI-STUDIES
IN CASES OF MUSCULOSKELETAL TUMORS

1. GENERAL CONSIDERATIONS ABOUT MR-CONTRAST MEDIA

Gadolinium-DTPA, the contrast medium used in this study, is a complex of the paramagnetic element Gd^{3+} chelated with DTPA (diethylene-triamine-pentaacetate). The reason for this chelation is to lower the toxicity of Gd itself and to control metabolism and excretion of the metal (1).
Paramagnetic substances (like Gd^{3+}) are characterized by the presence of one ore more unpaired electrons, which are responsible for their paramagnetic properties. They act as MR-contrast media by influencing strongly the relaxation of neighbouring protons, i.e. they behave as small magnets, they produce strong local magnetic fields and hence, cause an increase in relaxation rate (resulting in a decrease of T1 and T2).

2. PERFORMED STUDIES WITH Gd-DTPA

Contrast studies were performed in 32 patients with bone and soft tissue tumors or mimicking conditions.
Children under the age of 12 years were excluded from this study.

All patients were informed of the nature of potential benefits and possible risks of the investigation. Written consent was always obtained. Gd-DTPA (Schering AG, Berlin) was used in all cases.

Contrast medium was administrated by slow intravenous injection (90 sec) at a dose of 0.2 ml/kg body weight.

In this phase III-study, beside for its diagnostic value, we looked also for concomitant symptoms, such as: pain, heat sensation, nausea, vomiting, dizziness, headache, tachycardia, bradycardia, arrhytmia, hypertension, hypotension, dyspnea, allergy-like skin symptoms and Quincke's edema.
In none of the 32 cases any of these symptoms occurred, consequently, no therapeutic measures were installed.

After performing T1- and T2-WI, again T1-WI were obtained 5 min after contrast injection in all 32 patients, using the same parameters. No dynamic studies (images obtained with different time delay) were done.
In each case we estimated the raise of SI after contrast injection (SI after − SI before contrast) on T1-WI.
Therefore, we used the semiquantitative appreciation of SI as described in the chapter 2.
Raise of SI was also compared with SI on native T2-WI.
Finally, we tried to find specific patterns of enhancement.

3. COMMENT ON RESULTS

1. According to the degree of enhancement, we distincted three groups: a first group with no or only minimal enhancement (< 1.5), a second group with intermediate enhancement (between 1.5 and 2.5) and finally, a third group with pronounced enhancement (> 2.5).(Table 20.1)

124

Table 20.1. Groups of musculoskeletal lesions according to various degree of enhancement after Gd-DTPA:

Group I: no enhancement (0):	Group II: moderate enhancement (> 1.5, < 2.5):	Group III: pronounced enhancement (> 2.5):
juvenile bone cyst cartilage cap of osteochondroma malignant fibrous histio- cytoma (after radiotherapy)	chondrosarcoma (3 cases) giant cell tumor (borderline type) osteolytic metastasis (2 cases) aggressive fibromatosis liposarcoma (grade II) stress fracture hemangioma (com- pressive type)	osteosarcoma (3 cases) liposarcoma (grade III) osteolytic metastatis (3 cases) hemangioma (compressive type)
minimal enhancement (< 1.5):		
osteoid osteoma (2 cases) osteomyelitis non ossifying fibroma osteoblastic metastasis immunocytoma Paget's disease giant cell tumor (conventional type)		

2. Secondly, we looked for specific *patterns of enhancement*. Six different enhancement patterns were defined:

1/ *No enhancement* was seen in an irradiated malignant fibrous histiocytoma, in the cartilage cap of an osteochondroma and in a juvenile bone cyst.

2/ *Uniform enhancement* was seen around a stress fracture and around an osteoid osteoma. A giant cell tumor also showed this type of enhancement (Fig. 20.1.a and b).

3/ *Ringlike enhancement* was observed in a liposarcoma and in malignant tumors with central necrosis (Fig. 20.1.c and d).

4/ *Ringlike enhancement with papillary aspect of the internal borders* was encountered in the soft tissue components of most malignant tumors (Fig. 20.1.e, f, g and h).

5/ A *cocarde-like pattern* with central enhancement was seen in a case of metastasis (Fig. 20.1.i and j).

6/ a *pleiomorphic pattern*, i.e. a mixture of pattern 1,2,3 and 4, was observed in pleiomorphic liposarcoma and rhabdomyosarcoma (Fig. 20.1.k and l).

In a great number of cases, overall enhancement was difficult to assess because different tumor components showed different degrees of enhancement. Detailed description of enhancement after injection of Gd-DTPA is given for all tumors in the corresponding chapters.

3. Finally, we made a *comparison between SI-raise on T1-WI after contrast injection and SI on native T2-WI*.
Exception made for three of 32 cases (a juvenile bone cyst, the cartilage cap of an osteochondroma and a fibrous histiocytoma after combined radio-chemotherapy) a marked parallellism between the two parameters was noted (Table 20.2). We presume that this may be explained by the cellularity and the extent of interstitial space of the lesions. Indeed, malignant tumors are generally hypercellular, causing high SI on T2-WI, and have also large interstitial spaces, responsible for the significant enhancement after Gd-DTPA.

Table 20.2: **MR-grey scale of contrast enhancement**

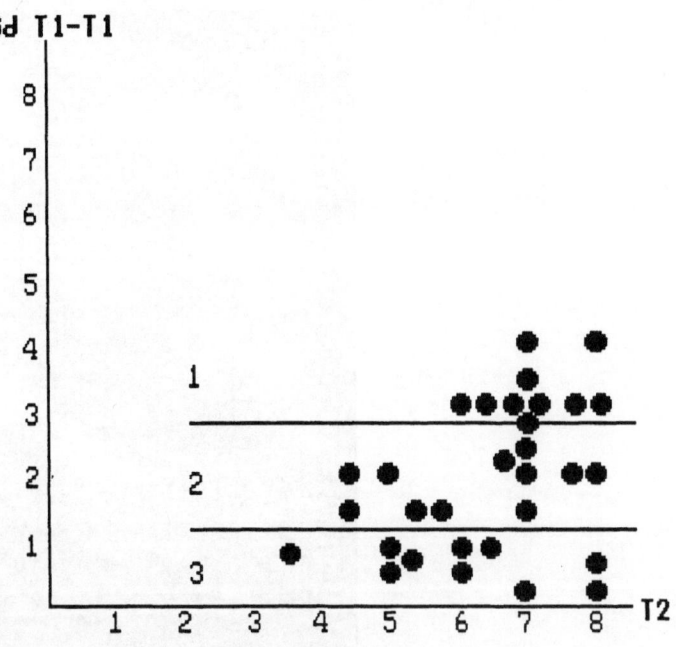

References

1. Roux E, De Broe L.Contrast agents in magnetic resonance imaging. JBR-BTR 1988; 1: 31-36.
2. Reiser M, Bohndorf K, Niendorf HP, et al. Erste Erfahrungen mit Gadolinium DTPA in der Magnetischen Resonanztomographie (MR) von Knochen- und Weichteiltumoren. Radiologe 1987; 27: 467-472.

126

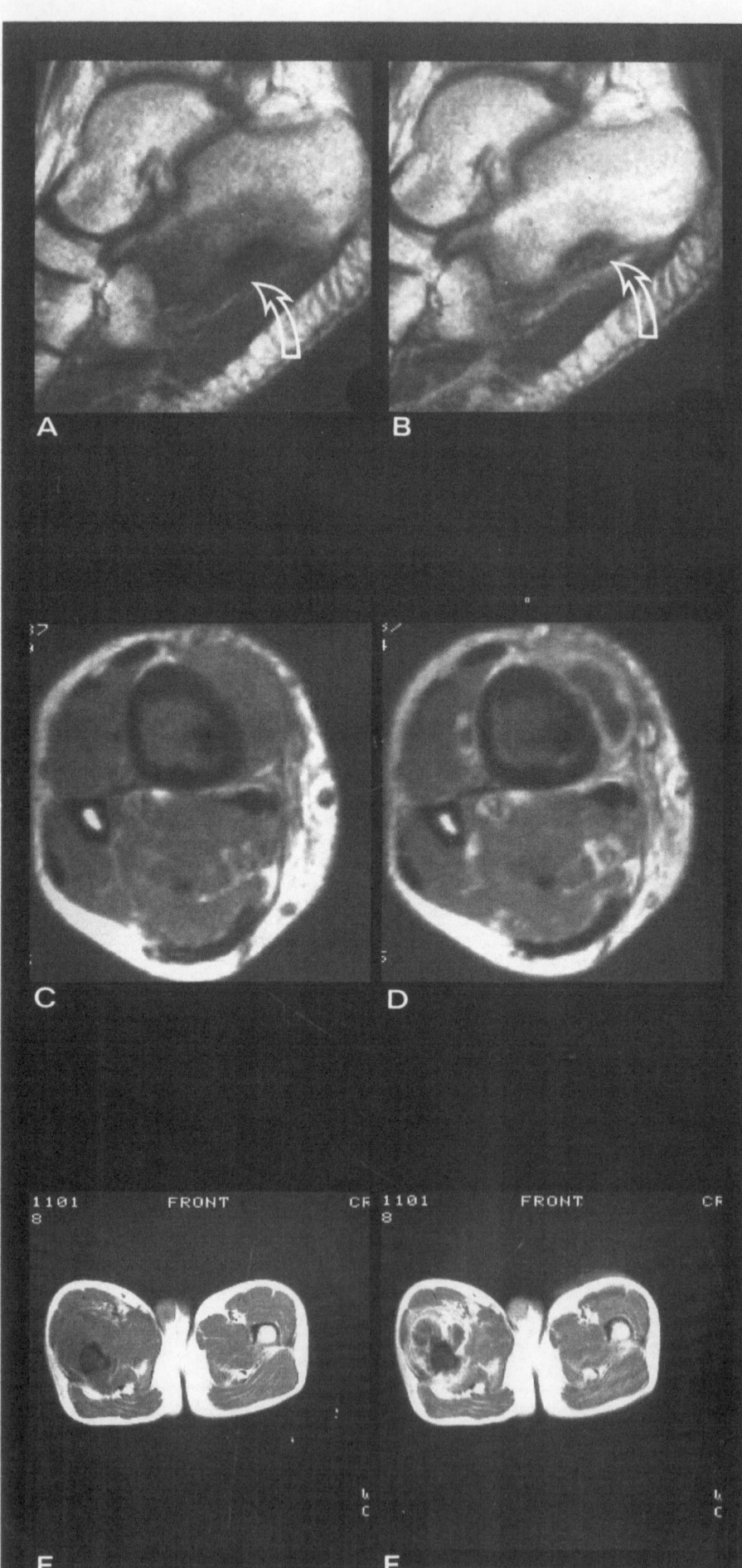

Fig.20.1. Patterns of enhancement after intravenous injection of Gd-DTPA.

20.1.a and b. Type II of enhancement in a case of osteoid osteoma (curved arrows) with edema of the surrounding bone marrow.
a. Region of decreased SI surrounding an osteoid osteoma.
b. Homogeneous enhancement of the medullary lesion which becomes less obvious after contrast injection.
20.1.c and d. Type III of enhancement in a case of chondrosarcoma with parosteal soft tissue involvement.
c. Parosteal soft tissue mass with SI of muscle [3].
d. Definite, ringlike enhancement at the periphery of the soft tissue mass after contrast injection.
20.1.e and f. Type IV of enhancement in a case of osteosarcoma with parosteal soft tissue mass.
e. Decreased SI at the medullary cavity. Large concentric parosteal mass with SI comparable with that of muscle [3].
f. Peripheral, papillary-like enhancement with unchanged SI of the central areas after contrast injection.

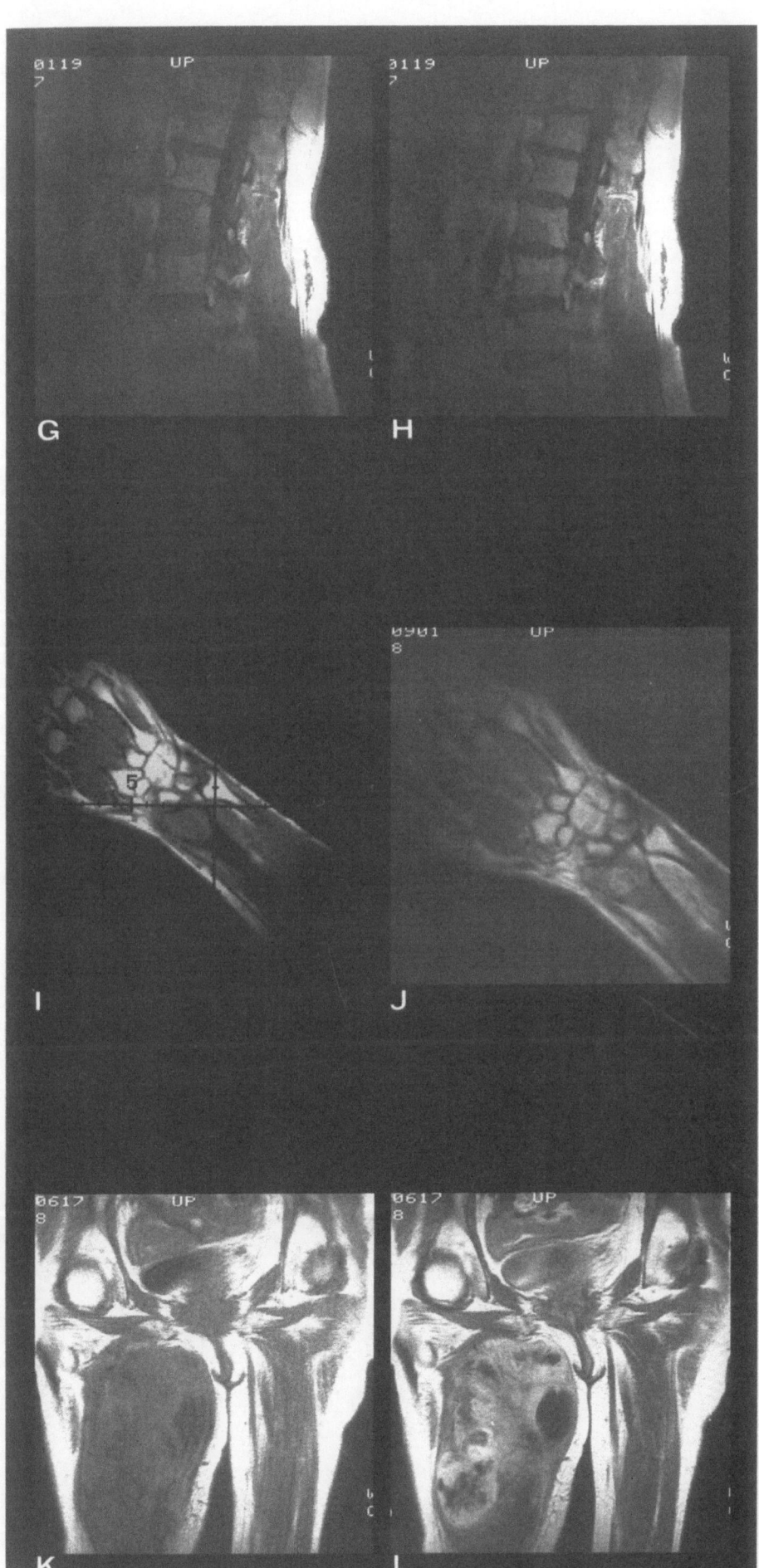

20.1.g and h. Type IV of enhancement
in a case of vertebral metastasis.
g. Decreased SI of the vertebral body
L III.
h. 'Filling in' phenomenon after contrast
injection.
20.1.i and j. Type V of enhancement in
a case of metastasis (primary tumor
unknown).
i. Intermediate SI [4] of the metastatic
lesion at the distal epi-metaphysis of
the left radius.
j. Central focus of intense enhancement
after contrast injection.
20.1.k and l. Type VI of enhancement in
a case of pleiomorphic
rhabdomyosarcoma.
k. Large tumoral mass with
inhomogeneous SI in the right thigh.
l. Pleiomorphic enhancement after
contrast injection.
Presence of areas of homogeneous,
papillary-like, ringlike and no
enhancement in the same lesion.

CHAPTER 21

GENERAL CONCLUSIONS

As 275 new cases of musculoskeletal neoplasms were collected in a period of 17 months among the 1 200 000 inhabitants of the province of Antwerp, this relatively high number reflects the importance of the subject being discussed.

Furthermore, since 94 of these patients underwent MRI, an assessment of the relative value of this imaging modality with respect to the treated subject is justified.

However, as for all imaging technologies, evaluation of the usefulness of MRI in the diagnostic work-up of musculoskeletal neoplasms is not only made by assessment of imaging and diagnostic efficacy, expressed in terms of sensitivity, specificity and overall accuracy, but should also include an evaluation of the patient's outcome and a cost-effectiveness assessment. Already patient's outcome is positively influenced by the complete non-invasive nature of the MRI-examination. Since the economic impact of MRI is beyond the scope of this study, considerations about cost-effectiveness cannot be further discussed in this monography.

As a consequence of the excellence of current available imaging techniques, including CR and CT, the prerequisites for MRI to become a valuable tool in the diagnostic work-up of bone and soft tissue neoplasms are very high. Diagnostic efficacy is determined by the effect of MRI on detection, characterization and evaluation of extent (staging) of musculoskeletal tumors. In spite of its outstanding contrast resolution and its multiplanar imaging capability, being all superior to those of the other imaging modalities, it is clear that, at this moment, MRI is not the first choice procedure for detection of bone neoplasms. Main reasons for this are the already high accuracy of CR, CT and RNSC (improved by MRI in only a small absolute number of cases), economic considerations, poor availability of MR-equipment and the complexity of the MRI-examination.

Similarly, although the soft tissue contrast obtained by MRI is definitely higher compared to that by other imaging modalities, making MRI extremely sensitive in demonstrating soft tissue neoplasms, MRI can neither be recommended yet as screening method for these tumors.

As a result of its high soft tissue contrast resolution, MRI is a highly valuable method for follow-up and detection of recurrence of tumor after surgery.

Definite characterization of musculoskeletal neoplasms by MRI is possible in a great number of cases. This number increases if the data from CR, CT and RNSC also are considered.

In some cases, a specific diagnosis was obtained by uniquely considering the SI of the lesions. This is shown in cases of bone cyst (by demonstrating fluid characteristics of tumor content), lipoma (fat content), non aggressive hemangioma (high SI on T1-WI), fibrosis (low SI both on T1- and T2-WI) and fibrous dysplasia (homogeneously distributed, intermediate SI, 'ground glass appearance').

Most commonly, however, a refinement of the differential diagnosis is obtained by combining morphological MRI-data with SI-characteristics. This is obvious in cases of chondrosarcoma (by showing lobules of very high SI on T2-WI), aneurysmal bone cyst (fluid-fluid levels), osteoid osteoma (bull's eye appearance).

The use of contrast media further improves specificity of the MRI-examination, by considering both degree and pattern of enhancement.

Finally, MRI-findings may indirectly improve diagnostic accuracy by serving as guide for the selection of an appropriate biopsy site.

The most constant improvement by MRI throughout the series of presented cases was obtained in determining the extent of the bone or soft tissue neoplasm.

Although an exact evaluation of this potential of MRI can only be assessed by comparing MRI-findings with those of macro- and micromorphologic studies of resected specimens, which were not always available as a consequence of modern conservative surgery, our findings as well as literature data suggest an accurate staging capability of MRI. With MRI both intraosseous and extraosseous extent, neurovascular involvement and joint involvement by bone and soft tissue tumors are easily evaluated. This results both from its very high contrast resolution and its multiplanar imaging capability and is extremely important as new conservative treatment procedures, such as conservative surgery, extracorporeal radiotherapy or sterilization, chemotherapy, ea. are more frequently applied.

As mentioned in the introductory chapter, two basic goals of the study have been achieved: firstly, providing an atlas of primary bone and soft tissue tumors and major mimics, that may serve as a guide for forthcoming cases, and, secondly, improving specificity of MRI-characteristics of primary musculoskeletal neoplasms by applying a more refined grey-scale of SI and by using paramagnetic contrast media.

In conclusion, despite the enormous potential of MRI, it is clear that, even with the advent of MRI, the imaging-pathological confrontation remains essential for an accurate diagnosis.

This was proved already in the first weeks after the end of the study. In a case of a soft tissue mass, MRI-features were highly suggestive of a chondrosarcoma, while histology only revealed myositis ossificans. A second look histology, however, revealed abnormal chondrocytes, suggesting a chondrosarcoma. Otherwise, a tumoral lesion in the left acetabular bone of a young boy presented with the charcteristics of a chondromatous tumor, i.e. lobulated formations with high SI on T2-WI. In contrast, pathologic examination of the resected specimen revealed an eosinophilic granuloma.

These cases also demonstrate that, while detection and staging no longer represent a challenge for medical imaging but have become reality, the confrontation imaging-pathology still remains the best procedure for the diagnosis of bone and soft tissue neoplasms.

(B 3291)
Brusselse straat 153 B-3000 Leuven
A. Struyf Oude Baan 353 B-3000 Leuven